BATH BOMBS
BALNEOTHERAPY

The Surprising Health Benefits of Bath Bombs & Ancient Secrets of Hot Springs, Dead Sea Minerals & Carbon Dioxide Baths

Mark Sloan

A proud presentation of:

ENDALLDISEASE.COM

ENDALLDISEASE
PUBLISHING

Published by Endalldisease Publishing
ISBN (kindle): 978-1-7772396-1-9
ISBN (paperback): 978-1-7772396-0-2
ISBN (audiobook): 978-1-7772396-2-6

Dedicated to my cat Meiko, who died during the writing of this book.

DISCLAIMER

This book does not claim or intend to treat, cure, heal, assess or reverse a disease, addiction, ailment, defect, injury or psychological condition. The information contained within this book should not be used to diagnose, treat or cure any medical condition, illness, disease, metabolic disorder or health problem of any kind. The information presented herein is for educational purposes only and is not intended as medical advice. If you have a medical problem, or suspect you have one, contact your physician or health care provider. Also, be sure to consult your physician or health care provider before beginning any kind of nutritional or exercise program. Neither the author nor the publisher assumes any liability for any injury, illness or adverse effects caused by the use or misuse of the information contained herein. Under no circumstances will any legal responsibility or blame be held against the publisher or author for any reparation, damages, or monetary loss due to the information in this book, either directly or indirectly. The reader is solely responsible for the use of the programs, advice and other information contained in this book.

TABLE OF CONTENTS

INTRODUCTION

If you're reading these words, you probably love indulging in warm, soothing baths and are captivated by the idea suggested in the title of this book – that every time you enjoy one of your favorite fizzy bath bomb treats, you are simultaneously doing something remarkably beneficial for your health.

Either that or you loved this book's flashy cover. (Don't you know you're not supposed to judge a book by its cover!!??) By doing so, you could end up buying a book that looks good on the outside, but its contents are just plain useless. Fortunately, this is not one of those books. It contains both a beautifully designed cover (thank you, Zeljka) and information inside that will forever change the way you look at taking a bath. The fact that you've purchased this book and are reading it now means you've already won. All that's left is to collect your hypothetical bag of gold coins and other informational gems in the pages to come.

Now seems like a good time to introduce myself. My name is Mark Sloan, and for the past 15 years, I have been obsessed with reading and researching every aspect of health that I could get my hands on. My obsession has been about trying to get well after the extreme trauma of losing my mother to cancer when I was 12 years old. One day she was here, the next, she was gone. People told me I lost my biggest fan at one of the most vulnerable parts of a young boy's life. But I didn't know any different. I carried on the best way I knew how like we all do when faced with tragedy. That's life, isn't it?

Anyway, my mother's death ultimately motivated me to read hundreds of books on nutrition, physiology, immunity, cellular biology, endocrinology, and many other fancy words that comprise the many systems of the body and factors pertaining to health. I ended up spending three years writing two books on Cancer, trying to figure out what this disease is and how to solve it. One of my goals before I leave this world is to make sure that no child will have to go through what I did – losing a parent to cancer – ever again.

While writing my books on cancer, I read literally thousands of different scientific and clinical studies and ended up referencing over 2,500 of them in the completed work. You can judge for yourself if you think I hit the nail on the head when you read my books *The Cancer Industry* and *Cancer: The Metabolic Disease Unravelled*, but I truly believe that these works have significantly advanced humanity's understanding of cancer – and most importantly, made it absolutely clear that nobody needs to die of cancer anymore. All the research needed to put the disease of cancer behind us forever has already been completed and, for the first time ever, is contained in two highly scientific yet simple-to-understand volumes. By the way, if you breathe air, then you need to read those books. But enough about that.

If it weren't for my mother's untimely death, I wouldn't have become the man I am today with all the opportunities I have to write books like this one. Instead of feeling sorry for myself and living life like a helpless victim, I used the pain inside me as motivation to create something that would ultimately save lives and change the world. See how this works? There's a bright side to everything – and you, too, can overcome tragedy in your life by seeing it as an opportunity and then taking massive action. But as much as I enjoy helping people create for themselves a meaningful existence, this is way outside the scope of this book. We're talking about bath bombs and balneotherapy here.

Discovery

Inspired by Alka-Seltzer tablets, the bath bomb was invented in 1989 by Lush Co-founder Mo Constantine in Dorset, England. Little did she know while working in her garden shed one day that she would invent a product that would go on to change the world of bathing forever. The original name given to the product before it was renamed to bath bomb was "Aqua sizzler."

In an article on Lush, the author explains the impact the bath bomb has had on the world since then, "Thirty years on, the bath bomb has evolved into a worldwide phenomenon, and is an established addition to any bathing ritual. From show stopping kaleidoscopes of colour, whizzing wonders that brighten and uplift, and softening soothers that help calm and relax, bath bombs have delighted and inspired millions, fought for peace and change, and bought about a cosmetic revolution from which there's no turning back."

"Everything you see today with the bath bombs has been evolved considerably from scratch," explains Mo, co-founder and inventor of the bath bomb. "It's madness really."

As revolutionary as the invention of the bath bomb is, we must give credit where credit is due and admit that it would be *nothing* without the bath. A bath bomb is simply one thing you can add to a bath to considerably enhance your bathing experience. As you're about to find out, this book is about far more than just bath bombs. Prepare yourself for an adventure into the amazing world of balneotherapy, which I'll introduce to you now.

The word *bath* comes from the Latin word *balneum*, and using baths therapeutically is called *Balneotherapy*. In the coming chapters, we are going to look at the lively history of therapeutic baths and how they have served to benefit the health of people for millennia. This will help give you an understanding of the value of warm mineral baths even before you drop in a sizzler.

But in order to truly understand what baths can do for your health, you must first have a basic understanding about your body's metabolism. I've dedicated an entire chapter to the subject of metabolism and will return to it at various other points in the book to show you how everything relates. As you're about to find out, maintaining a high metabolism is the number one most important thing you can do to improve your health.

When it comes to bathing in hot springs, salty seas, or bath tubs, there are a number of properties contained within the water that bestow therapeutic properties. We're going to look in depth at properties like carbonation, mineral content, and temperature, as well as their impact on metabolic rate.

I'll also present to you some of the beautiful and therapeutic naturally carbonated hot springs that exist in the world and how the water within these contain some of the same properties that a bath bomb infuses into a bath tub. But here's a fair warning: this book will probably inspire you to add many new bullet points to your bucket list of places to visit before your time is up. However, thanks to the bath bomb and the availability of ocean mineral salts, there's no reason to wait for vacation time to gain the benefits of bathing in a natural spring. After you understand the nourishing environment that bath bombs and other ingredients dissolved in water can create, you might begin storing your bath supplies in the medicine cabinet instead of next to that old, stinky toothbrush beneath your sink.

But how could a colorful, fizzy round ball of powder dunked in water possibly bestow such robust benefits? Like students on Miss Frizzle's magic school bus, we will go on a field trip inside the human body to help you understand how the primary active ingredient in bath bombs positively interacts with the physiology of every cell, every organ, and every tissue in your body.

The major goals of this book are simple...

1. To show you that learning can be fun and exciting. I hope this book ignites a passion inside you that may have been extinguished by the long, boring days spent in school learning impractical things.

2. To make you even more excited about baths by showing you that adding a sizzling bath bomb to your nightly soak in the tub is

doing far more good for your health and wellbeing than just stimulating your senses with some fizz, color, and flowery aromas.

3. To put balneotherapy back on the map – for you and for society as a whole – as one of the most valuable forms of therapy ever discovered.

4. To determine the ultimate healing bath formulation; which ingredients can be added to a bath to create the most therapeutic therapeutic bathing environment possible.

Yes, I want to change the way you think about baths – from a relaxing activity to a powerful therapeutic modality – and to get you to associate a bath bomb-infused bath with one of the first line of therapies you should reach for next time you are ill.

This book has the potential to radically improve your health and enhance the quality of your life. Virtually every organ and system of your body can benefit from the medicinal properties of a bath bomb bath. I know, I know. You're so excited right now that your hands are shaking. Mine are too! But that's because I'm on my third cup of coffee after many hours of writing. Speaking of writing, before we wrap up this intro, I want to say a few things about my writing style.

In my previous books I wrote on Cancer, for example, I had to take a fairly serious approach since it was a serious subject. My book *Red Light Therapy: Miracle Medicine* was written in a similar way. But after receiving feedback from readers for a couple of years, it turns out, much to my surprise, that most people don't appreciate having 100 pages of references at the end of a book – even if it is to back up everything I say with scientific evidence. So, I've decided to cut back on the reference listings while at the same time remaining every bit as scientific as far as where the information was derived. But there's another major change that I'm striving to implement in my writing that will help me grow as a man and enhance your experience as a reader.

Stan Lee, the former head of Marvel Comics and co-creator of legendary characters like Spiderman, the Hulk, and the Fantastic Four once said, "If you have a character that seems to be all perfect, it's hard to relate to him because when you read a story, you really want to empathize with the character that you are reading about."

The last thing I want to do is come across as sterile or perfect and make it hard to empathize with me because I seem flawless and with no problems. As such, one of the things I've been most excited about in writing this book is the opportunity to broaden my literary horizons by communicating more of my personality, while at the same time delivering to you the most practical and life-changing information that I can.

The type of information with the greatest potential to improve our lives involve things that have been observed, tested, and repeated – because things that have been observed, tested, and repeated are as close to truth as we can get. My job is to bring to light many of the great discoveries of scientists past, which have been buried in a thick layer of dust in scientific journals, so they can be used for your benefit and the benefit of all. After that, it's your job to put the information into practice and see if it works for you.

Clear as mud? Excellent! Now, let's get started.

CHAPTER 1

HISTORY OF BALNEOTHERAPY

Balneotherapy is an ancient and traditional form of therapy in which you bathe in warm, mineral-rich, and sometimes carbonated spring water for better health.

There are many different words that are used to describe the therapeutic use of baths besides balneotherapy, including spa therapy, mineral baths, hydropathy, hydrotherapy, water therapy, aquatic therapy, and pool therapy. Whichever term you prefer, they all involve submerging the body in *water*.

Therapeutic use of water is as old as mankind. It has been recorded in ancient Egypt, Greek and Roman civilizations; it is steeped in thousands of years of Japanese tradition, and has been foundational for facilitating recovery and enhancing quality of life in virtually all world cultures throughout history.

"Water is without doubt the most ancient
of all remedial agents for disease."
— John Harvey Kellogg

The following statue depicts a man breaking a walking crutch – an eloquent symbol of balneotherapy – in the ancient spa town of Piešťany, Slovakia.

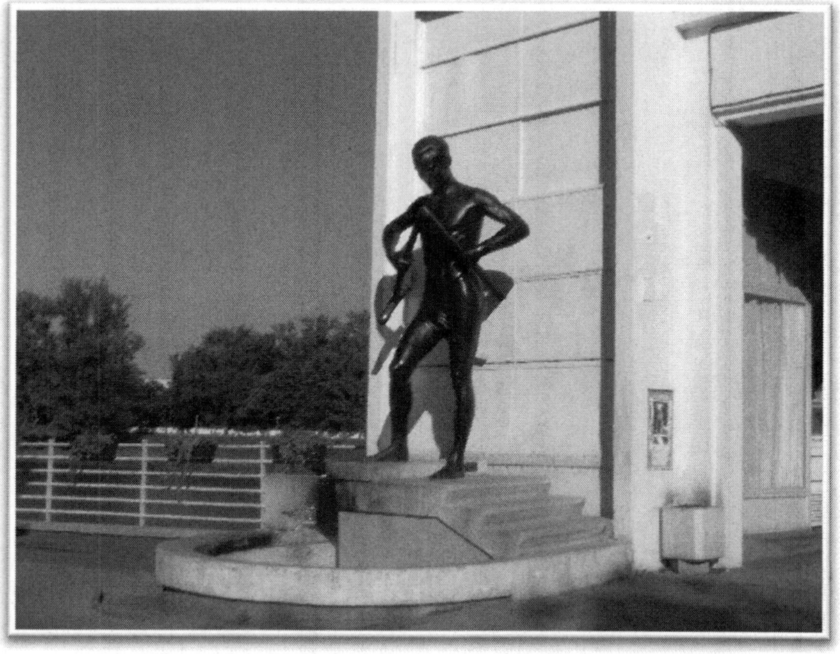

Image: A statue of a man breaking his walking crutch in Slovakia reveals the virtues of balneotherapy.

This work of art testifies to the amazing therapeutic value that balneotherapy bestows upon the people of Piešťany and its significance in their lives.

Greece

Ancient Greeks used spas and mineral waters for therapy and to keep fit. Greek mythology is rich in legends linked with spring waters and Greek gods and goddesses. For example, Venus, the goddess of beauty, who bathed in her temple with the assistance of her maidservants, or Ira, the mother of Gods, who bathed in a spring once a year to restore her virginity.

Many people know that Hippocrates, the founder of modern medicine, was a big proponent of food as medicine. What most people don't know is that he also routinely prescribed balneotherapy in mineral spring water to his sick patients.

"He, who wishes to practice good medicine,
must be conversant with the following:
First, and finally, one should be aware of the
power of waters; because as they vary in taste and
origin, their healing power may vary as well."
— Hippocrates

Italy

It was the Greeks who introduced balneotherapy to the Romans. In ancient Rome, scattered about the city were large imperial bath complexes called *Thermae*, which were open and freely available for public use. These luxurious public bathing facilities were used as a place for therapy and relaxation, but they also served as meeting places, centers of entertainment, culture, gymnastics, art, debate, and cleansing. Roman bath establishments effectively enabled the building and strengthening of relationships and community.

Spain

Treatments combining the use of mineral-rich seawater with sunshine therapy have been in use in Spain since the Roman Empire, according to Dr. Elena Ledo in her paper titled *Mineral Water and Spas in Spain*. Today, there are over 300 spas in Spain, or one balneotherapy facility for every 130,000 people.

Korea

In 1458, Korean King Sejong of the Lee Dynasty allegedly cured his chronic skin disease by bathing in the thermal waters of what is known today as Onyang Spa. King Sejong erected a monument at the spa which remains to this day. There are currently more than 20 spas in Korea, according to Dr. Seung-Kyung Hann, the oldest being Dongnae Spa, whose waters have been used for arthritis since around 935 BC.

Poland

In Poland, the father of balneotherapy was Dr. Wojciech Oczko, a royal physician who wrote the first papers on the subject in the 16th century. To this day, balneotherapy exerts a strong influence over the medical field in Poland. Doctors are taught courses on balneotherapy during their medical education, and balneotherapy is commonly used as a supplement to pharmacotherapy on patients, according to a paper by Drs. Omulecki, Nowak and Zalewska.

Bulgaria

In Bulgaria, use of mineral springs and spas also dates back to antiquity. Most of the larger cities in Bulgaria actually began as spa resorts before becoming larger population centers, in as early as the first century BC. Many of these spa resorts are still active today for recreational and medical purposes.

"The vital, colorful, and often exotic atmosphere of Bulgarian spas inspires the visitors to understand the folklore and experience the hospitality of the warm-hearted Bulgarian people"

— Dr. Snejina Vasseileva

Israel

Israel boasts numerous resorts and curative balneotherapy centers that specialize in skin and musculoskeletal disorders. The most famous place to receive balneotherapy potentially in the world is the Dead Sea in Israel. You'll learn all about it soon. Israel's hot mineral springs offer a natural approach for skin and inflammatory diseases, utilizing sunshine, balneotherapy, and mud in a calm, pleasant environment.

France

France is home to the world-renowned thermal spa La Roche-Posay, whose mineral waters have been known and used medically for over 1700 years. Although La Roche-Posay mineral waters contain an overall low concentration of minerals, its unique water properties contain the essential element selenium. Due to soil depletion, people who don't eat enough seafood are probably deficient in selenium and could benefit from balneotherapy at La Roche-Posay. Every year, thousands of patients suffering from atopic dermatitis, psoriasis, burns, ichthyosis, keratodermias, rosacea, and severe acne are doctored at La Roche-Posay Spa.

Portugal

Mineral waters and spas have been used in what is modern day Portugal for centuries. In many parts of Portugal, ruins of large Roman Baths can be seen, including some built as long ago as 49 BC under the order of Julius Caesar. The founder of the country of Portugal, D. Afonso Henriques (1143), after being wounded in the battle of Badajoz, spent some time in the spa of S. Pedro do Sul. More than 500 years ago, Europe's oldest thermal hospital was built at the hot mineral springs of Caldas da Rainha, which is still in use to this day. While the hospital at Caldas da Rainha traditionally used only water therapies, today it uses a combination of water and modern medical treatments.

The Many Approaches to Balneotherapy

Balneotherapy can involve a broad range of approaches that adjust certain properties of the water including temperature (hot or cold), mineral content, and some can even alter the water pressure. Others utilize water jets, massages, floatation tanks, and of course, the addition of bath bombs.

We'll take a much closer look at the effects of temperature on your health in a future chapter, but for now, I'll introduce you to some of the fascinating accounts of people who use cold water therapeutically.

What's Cooler Than Being Cold?

Certain Olympic athletes, like gold medal swimmer Michael Phelps, as well as athletes in a variety of professional sports, soak in *ice baths* following intense exercise and competition to help speed up bodily recovery.

After winning the 10,000m event at the 2002 European championships, gold medal marathon runner Paula Radcliffe attributed her victory to her soaking in ice cold water. "It's absolute agony, and I dread it, but it allows my body to recover so much more quickly," said Radcliffe.

In addition to sports, ice baths have also been used as a part of military training.

Dutch extreme athlete Wim Hof is noted for his ability to withstand freezing temperatures and he has set world records for swimming under ice, for prolonged contact with ice, and for running a half-marathon barefoot on snow and ice. All of these extraordinary feats he ascribes to what he called the *Wim Hof Method*, which is a regimen involving three pillars:

1. Cold therapy
2. Breathing
3. Meditation

The water portion of his regimen is the cold therapy, which ranges from exposing oneself to cold water at the end of a shower, to regular ice baths for more experienced practitioners.

The evidence indicating that a quick dunk in frigid water is beneficial is vast and well established. Cold thermogenesis, or the stimulation of the body's metabolism by a quick dunk in frigid waters, has been measured in humans as early as 1780 by Antoine Lavoisier. The way it works is by stimulating the production of heat in the body in order to maintain a stable core body temperature. That increase in temperature, is regulated by thyroid hormone, so a quick boost in thyroid function is the mechanism of action of this form of water therapy. Research has shown that cold thermogenesis can increase human metabolism by up to 280%.

Every morning, motivational speaker and life coach Tony Robbins jumps into his frigid 57-degree 4'x4' plunge pool as a way to induce thermogenesis, and also, to overcome mental resistance and show his mind who is boss. By consciously doing something uncomfortable that your mind most certainly objects to, you gain a greater degree of control over your ability to take action and accomplish goals and other difficult tasks. That's the idea.

Here's a link to a video of Tony taking the plunge: https://www.youtube.com/watch?v=x9g6O7Y6bks

But enough of all this cold water body and mind mastery! Let's do a cannon ball in the hot tub.

Three Basic Approaches to Balneotherapy

There are basically three main ways to obtain balneotherapy – by bathing in a sea or ocean, in a natural spring, or in a bath tub. One of the best things about receiving therapy in the salty ocean or in a natural hot spring is that these therapies don't cost you a dime. People regularly pay top dollar to receive similar treatments at a spa, and when you run a hot bath at home, you pay for the water, for the fuel to heat that water, and for the minerals and other ingredients you add to it. Some of the best things in life *truly are* free.

Anyway, we'll cover oceans and seas more in depth in a future chapter. Right now I want to focus on hot springs: what they are, where they're located, and their medicinal potential.

Natural Hot Springs

A hot spring, sometimes called a hydrothermal spring or a geothermal spring, is a spring produced when geothermally heated groundwater squeezes through cracks in the bedrock on its way up to the earth's surface.

Every single continent in the world contains hot springs, and they are prevalent in some countries more than others. Countries renowned for hot springs include Honduras, Canada, Chile, China, Costa Rica, Hungary, Iceland, Iran, Israel, Japan, New Zealand, Peru, Romania, Taiwan, Turkey, Fiji, and the United States. Surrounding some of these hot springs is natural scenery of breathtaking beauty, like many of the ones in Japan, for example – but I doubt there's a hot spring experience that you would not consider beautiful.

This list of hot springs is a valuable resource for finding a hot spring near you: https://en.wikipedia.org/wiki/List_of_hot_springs

Take note that although the list of hot springs on that page is lengthy, it doesn't contain every hot spring in the world. Together we can make it better: if you know of a hot spring that's not in this list, go ahead and add it.

The water in many hot springs is somewhere around 100 degrees, which is perfect for bathing. However, some hot springs are far too hot to immerse yourself in and could result in burns or even death – if, for some reason, you decided to ignore the steam burns to your skin and eyes that you got while approaching the extremely hot water and jumped in anyway. Seriously though, hot springs located in volcanic areas are often at or near boiling point, and some people have been scalded or even killed by entering these springs, whether intentionally or by accident.

If you value your life, a good example of a hot spring you would never want to bathe in – but also arguably one of the most beautiful hot springs you'll ever see – is the Grand Prismatic Spring in Yellowstone National Park, USA. It is the largest hot spring in the United States and the third-largest in the entire world, after Frying Pan Lake in New Zealand and Boiling Lake in Dominica. This spring is 160° F, so bring some raw milk if you prefer drinking it pasteurized, but please do not bathe in this colorful, alien-looking washbasin of death!!

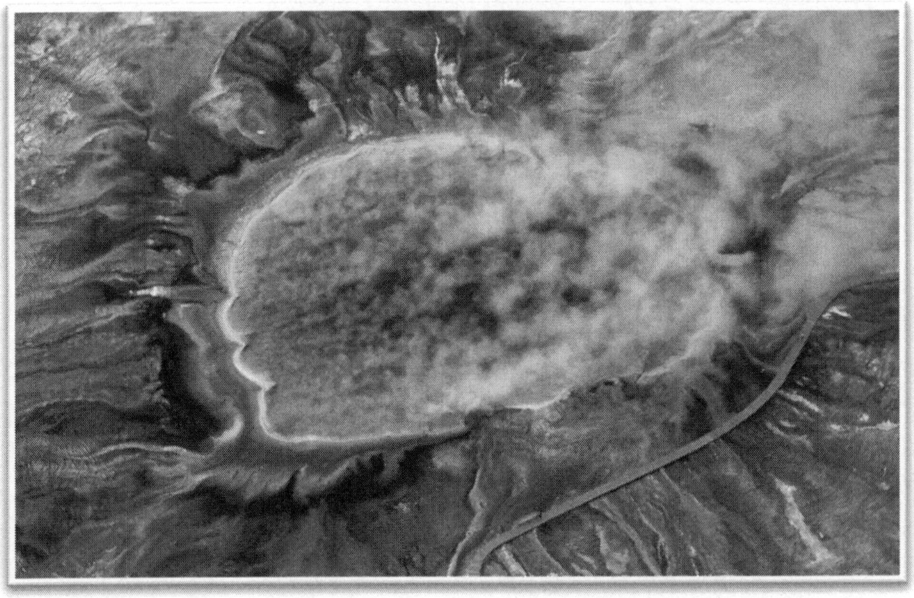

Image: The Grand Prismatic Spring in Yellowstone National Park

In addition to temperature, other factors believed to contribute to the rejuvenation imparted by balneotherapy include the water's mineral content as well as its carbon dioxide content. We will explore each of these factors in great detail in their individual chapters as we make our way through this ~~book~~ adventure on balneotherapy.

The Rise and Fall of Balneotherapy in the US

Around the year 1835, there was a massive upsurge in the medical use of balneotherapy in Western medicine, including the United States and Canada. In fact, most people will be surprised to hear that for the next 100 years, water therapy was literally the *primary therapy* for all ailments. At the peak of popularity in the United States, there were over

200 water therapy clinics, most located in the Northeast. These clinics also sprouted up in many European countries. Some of the famous patients treated at a hydrotherapy clinic in Malvern, England include Charles Darwin, Charles Dickens, Thomas Carlyle, Florence Nightingale, Lord Tennyson, and Samuel Wilberforce.

Unfortunately, this golden era of aquatic medicine didn't last. Despite its widespread acceptance and popularity, around the year 1950, medical use of balneotherapy in Western medicine vanished practically overnight.

Why did balneotherapy vanish from Western medicine so abruptly and completely?

Unfortunately, we can never know for sure, but the change probably had something to do with powerful individuals wanting to replace the unprofitable water therapy industry with the colossal $3.4 Trillion drug- and surgical-based medical behemoth that we have today.

Balneotherapy is 'Quackery'?

Today, despite thousands of years of balneotherapy use all over the world, balneotherapy is not taken seriously in Western medicine. In fact, try telling your doctor you wish to try bathing instead of the bottle of drugs she prescribed you and she will probably laugh in your face. People tend to think of the spa as a place of recreation where they can go for the day to get pampered and beautified in a relaxing environment. But the spa is far more than that.

It's time to teach the world what people have known since time immemorial: that the benefits of wading in warm, salty water can be miraculous.

This book represents the resuscitation and revival of an ancient therapeutic modality whose potential is so vast, that its return as a foundational remedy in medicine is inevitable.

I just had a good thought while writing this: every day on the radio, the TV news, in music and in movies, we are constantly bombarded with stories that remind us of our differences. Imagine for a second what life could be like without all these walls put up between people of different ages, sexes, cultures, countries, religions, etc. What better way to make that happen than to hold as our highest value bathing, like the Romans and so many other cultures of the past? Its ability to promote wellness and build community is unmatched. Because who doesn't love a hot bath? NOBODY!

So maybe for your next family vacation you could spend a week soaking together at a beautiful and relaxing hot spring resort like Cascate del Mulino in Italy, Hotel Matumotoro in Japan, or the Blue Lagoon in Iceland.

Here's what your family photo will look like...

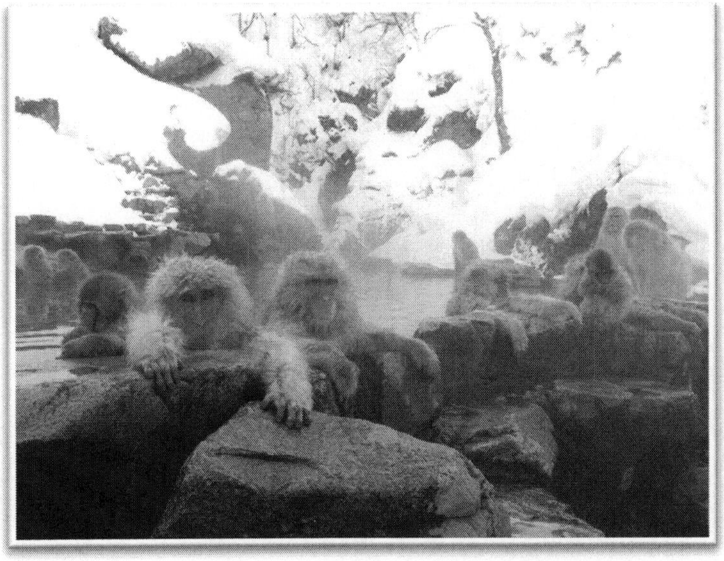

Image: Macaques enjoying an open air hot spring in Nagano, Japan.

After daily indulgences in the Laugarvatn hot spring in Iceland with the local people of all ages for an entire month, writer and co-founder of *Siren Magazine* Raisa Imogen wrote, "What a crazy miracle that warm water bubbles up from the frozen ground in the midst of winter! And has been doing so for thousands and thousands of years. It is a powerful reminder for me that sometimes, what is most nourishing and beautiful runs underneath the surface of what seems cold and hard."

CHAPTER 2

METABOLISM & THE ROOT CAUSE OF DISEASE

Currently there are over 30,000 officially classified diseases in the medical world. This is convenient and profitable for the medical industry because they can produce and market at least one new drug for every disease. But the reality is there aren't 30,000 diseases.

The truth, always simple and beautiful, is there's only one disease: either your cells are functioning properly or they're not. When a group of cells malfunction, they will begin to cause symptoms in the body, which your doctor will use to diagnose you with a disease. But that disease is just a name; it doesn't exist. What does exist is your body, which is nothing but a collection of cells – and if you're sick, your cells have simply stopped doing what they're supposed to do.

What is it that cells are supposed to do that causes disease when they fail to do it? In one word: metabolism.

Many people when they think of the word metabolism, they think weight loss. And while it's true that increasing metabolism is the best way to shed excess pounds, the significance of having a high metabolism goes far beyond just losing weight. Put simply, metabolism can be defined as the amount of energy the cells of your body produces at rest in a given period of time.

When you're born, your metabolism is at its highest, and then throughout life, it will gradually decrease all the way up until your point of death. In most cases, a newborn baby is the epitome of health, and its high metabolic rate will usually continue this way throughout childhood, as indicated by their ability to bounce off walls with a seemingly endless supply of energy. Every year, the metabolism will slowly and gradually lose its efficiency until one day in old age when energy production runs out completely and they pass on.

A low metabolism can manifest itself in any number and combination of symptoms, but regardless of the "disease" name your doctor gives to your particular set of symptoms, what's happening is low metabolism.

"If we learn to see problems in terms of a general disorder of energy metabolism, we can begin to solve them."

— Dr. Ray Peat

When your metabolism is high, every organ and system of your body will function better than when your metabolism is low. Everything works better with a high metabolism.

Metabolism takes place inside every one of the trillions of cells that make up your body. A healthy cell will oxidize sugar within tiny organelles inside your cells called mitochondria, and an unhealthy cell will not.

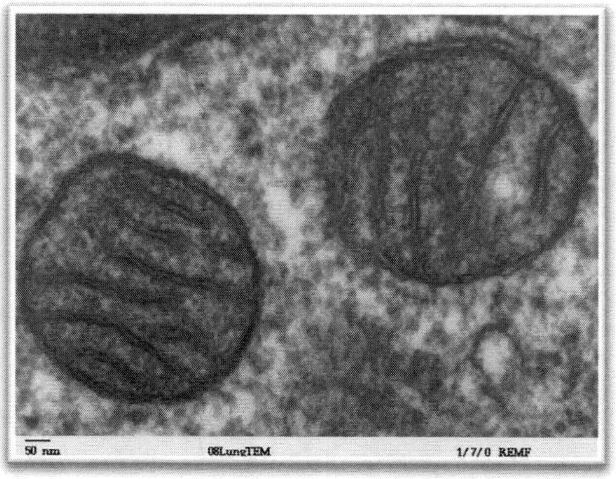

Image: Two mitochondria from mammalian lung tissue displaying their matrix and membranes as shown by electron microscopy

When functioning properly, energy is produced within the mitochondria of your cells and the process involves the breakdown of glucose by oxygen into the energy currency of your body known as adenosine triphosphate or ATP. Another very underappreciated and misunderstood product of mitochondrial metabolism is carbon dioxide. Medical students and anyone else learning about cellular metabolism in university are taught carbon dioxide is a 'waste product,' but nothing could be further from the truth. A high level of carbon dioxide in the body is evidence that your cells are metabolizing properly. CO2 keeps the metabolism humming by dilating blood vessels and shuttling oxygen into cells. Without adequate CO2, blood flow is stunted, oxygen use by cells halts, and your metabolism fails.

Some hot springs in the world are naturally carbonated with tiny bubbles of carbon dioxide like a soda pop. The carbon dioxide present in certain springs and baths is most likely the most beneficial ingredient in all of balneotherapy.

Author of the world's leading medical physiology textbook Dr. Arthur C. Guyton once said, "All chronic pain, suffering and disease are caused by a lack of oxygen at the cell level."

When cells lose their ability to use oxygen to breakdown and convert glucose into utilizable energy, overall health suffers.

We will get to many specific examples of diseases that can be resolved by increasing the metabolism in future chapters. In this chapter, I'll keep the examples to a minimum but give you a taste of the importance of proper metabolism for hair growth and the vitality of skin.

A 2018 experiment published in the journal *Nature* gives us a fascinating glimpse into what can happen when efficient metabolism within the mitochondria of cells is inhibited. When the scientists switched off mitochondrial function within cells of mice, they observed "profound effects on the skin resulting in wrinkles and visual hair loss with an increased number of dysfunctional hair follicles and inflammatory responses." Low metabolism resulted in wrinkles, hair loss, and also "markedly increased skin inflammation that appears to be a contributing factor in skin pathology." Remarkably, scientists reported that when mitochondrial function was restored, the wrinkles and hair loss *were reversed!*

The big message from this study is exactly what I've been saying repeatedly in this chapter: Restoring dysfunctional metabolism so that cells can produce energy efficiently within the mitochondria of cells is the most efficient approach to reversing all diseases and pathologies.

Now that you have a better understanding of the centrality of metabolism in health, the stage has been set for us to look at the impact of balneotherapy on metabolism.

The bath properties or ingredients that we're going to look at in relation to metabolism in the following chapters include:

- Temperature
- Minerals
- Carbonation

The purpose of these investigations will be, first and foremost, to help us better understand how our bodies function, but it will also be instrumental in our quest to find the ultimate bath recipe that we can use as a potent strategy to increase and maintain as high a metabolism as possible for the rest of our lives.

Temperature

What's more therapeutic: a cold spring or a hot spring? And is there one specific temperature that will provide maximum benefit?

Minerals

Does mineral-rich water confer more, less or the same therapeutic value as water without minerals? If the answer is mineral-rich water, then which mineral or combination of minerals has the greatest positive impact on metabolism?

Carbonation

What does carbon dioxide have to do with cellular oxygen use? And what effect does bathing in carbonated water have on cellular metabolism? Is there a way to add carbonation to my bath tub at home?

I know what you're thinking: *I thought this was a book on bath bombs – when are you going to talk about bath bombs!!??* Go jump in a hot spring and *relax*. I've dedicated an entire chapter to bath bombs, which we'll get to after I answer all the above questions in the next few chapters. Like cheese or a fine wine, the longer you wait, the better it will be.

Conclusions

There are over 30,000 officially named diseases in the world today, but the cause of all of them is the same: A malfunctioning cell.

The job of the cells in your body is to produce energy, in a process called metabolism. Biological energy is produced by your cells through the oxidation of glucose within your mitochondria.

It is enzymes that power the entire metabolic process, and if one single vitamin or mineral needed to produce your essential metabolic enzymes is not available, the enzyme will not be produced, your metabolism will malfunction, and your metabolic rate will fall.

The defining characteristic of a cell in metabolic disarray is that it has lost its ability to utilize oxygen, which, according to Dr. Guyton, is the root cause of all disease. Fix the disorder, and you fix the disease.

When your cells have everything they need to function properly, cellular metabolism will be efficient and your cells will be healthy. And when all the cells in your body are healthy, you will be healthy. This is why a high metabolic rate is the number one thing to focus on for improving health.

Key Points to Remember

- There is only one disease: A malfunctioning cell.
- Your body is a collection of cells, and if your cells are functioning properly, you are healthy.
- The job of your cells is to produce energy for your entire body, in a process called metabolism.
- When your metabolism is low, symptoms will eventually manifest – and to raise the metabolic rate is to fix the root cause of the symptoms.
- Restoring dysfunctional metabolism, so that cells can produce energy efficiently within the mitochondria of cells, is the most efficient approach to reversing all diseases and pathologies.

CHAPTER 3

TEMPERATURE

The use of springs and spas as medicine throughout history involved the immersion of people in both cold and hot water. While some doctors believed cold water was more valuable, others believed it was hot water that had greater medical value. Some doctors believed in both, and alternated patients back and forth between hot and cold water a number of times in a single session, which could be ideal.

In this chapter, we're going to determine whether bathing in hot or cold water – or both – has the greatest therapeutic effect.

Temperature and Metabolism

Immersing the body in cold or hot water can quickly change body temperature, which alters cellular metabolism in important ways. For example, would a T-bone steak decompose more quickly – or less quickly - if you left it on the counter at room temperature, compared to inside a fridge?

Of course, the answer is it would rot more quickly on the countertop – that's why refrigerators exist! The function of a fridge is to cool things down to slow the chemical and bacterial metabolic reactions that serve to decompose various foods.

The same accelerating or slowing of chemical reactions occurs when the body is exposed to hot or cold. This includes all the chemical reactions required for your metabolism to produce energy. In other words, if your core body temperature drops too low, your metabolic rate will slow down.

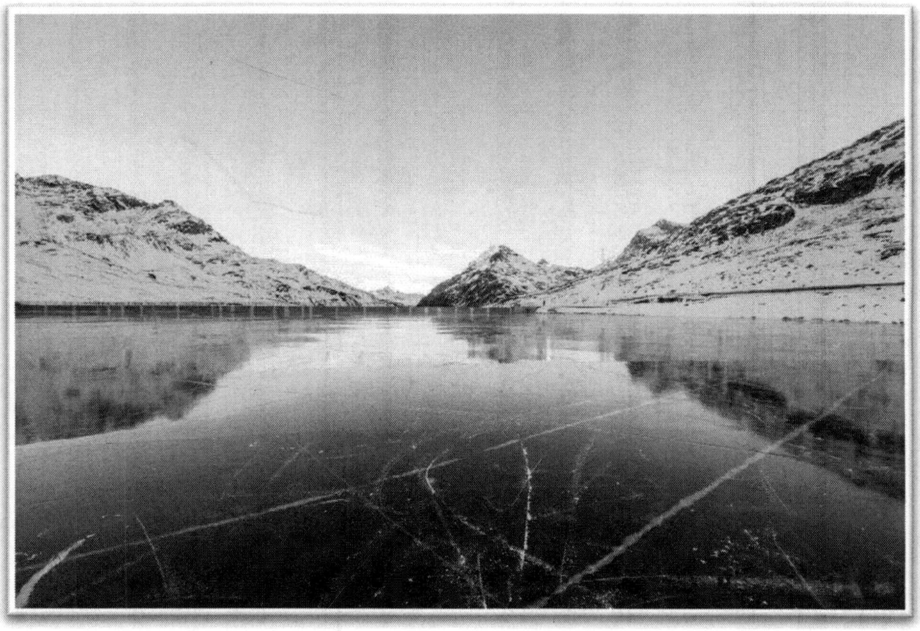

Cold Water Effects on Metabolism

As previously mentioned, remarkable metabolic enhancing effects have been reported after quick immersion in cold water. Submerging the body in cold water stimulates the metabolism by forcing the body to heat itself up. But when a person stays in cold water too long, the energy needed to warm the body back up runs out, and stress hormones are elevated to begin breaking down and consuming your own body tissues, including your muscles, brain and other organs, to use for energy instead.

In that state of elevated stress, where the body is actively breaking down soft tissues to use for energy to meet the demands of the stress caused by freezing temperatures, what do you think would happen if the body maintained a high rate of energy production (aka a high metabolic rate)?

That's right. The body would eat itself to death very quickly. That's why your body's response to all types of stressors is to reduce your metabolism as much as possible to prevent death by what is formally called cachexia. Oh and by the way, most cancer patients die of cachexia. It's the stress and its negative effects that kill cancer patients, not some kind of "werewolf" cancer cell.

In the short term, cold water immersion can bestow great therapeutic benefit. I suspect most people don't have access to two bath tubs side by side, but if you do, it's probably very beneficial to alternate between hot and cold multiple times, as many Western medical doctors did for patients in the 19th century. However, keep in mind that any prolonged soaking in cold water can dramatically lower your metabolism, so keep your cold water immersion quick, probably no longer than a minute or so each time.

Your Temperature Indicates Your Metabolic Rate

One of the most accurate indicators of your metabolic rate can be measured at home, anytime day or night, using a ten dollar thermometer from the drugstore.

The ideal body temperature is around 98.6° F. Having a temperature of 98.6° F, or slightly above throughout the day, is one of the most accurate indicators of a high metabolic rate.

Now that you know the secret, you can check the status of your health at any given time, and you also have a means to measure whether that new diet or exercise program you've been trying out is working or not. Measuring your temperature just before a meal, and then again 30 minutes after, is a good way to determine if your body is effectively digesting and assimilating those nutrients. If your temperature has increased, it means the nutrients in the food you ate are being absorbed and utilized metabolically. If your temperature has dropped, the meal has had a negative effect on your metabolic rate.

Worldwide Metabolic Rates in Decline

The metabolic rates of people worldwide over the past 100 years have been in a steady decline. So much so that an eerie article appeared in the *New York Times* in 2009 titled "Rethinking 98.6." Few people have a high metabolic rate these days, and as such, average body temperatures are lower than they've ever been.

To put into perspective what that means, the average body temperature of a bird is 105° F. That's a very high metabolic rate, and consider how much energy they expend flapping their wings while flying.

"The animal with the lowest metabolic rate in all of the animal kingdom is the sloth, with a resting body temperature as low as 86° F," wrote metabolism expert, health writer, and author Matt Sone. "Do a little research on the characteristics that define sloth-like behavior," Matt continued, "and you'll see some parallels to the changes humans experience when their metabolic rate falls."

I don't know about you, but I don't want energy levels to be in any way similar to that of a sloth – yet it was only about five years ago that my metabolism was as low as 94.5° F upon waking. It was no coincidence that I could barely get out of bed.

The key point to remember here is that your metabolic rate will drop in direct proportion to a reduction in your core body temperature.

Warm Water Effects on Metabolism

If your body temperature is low, any method you can use to raise it will help reduce the stress your body is under and raise your metabolism.

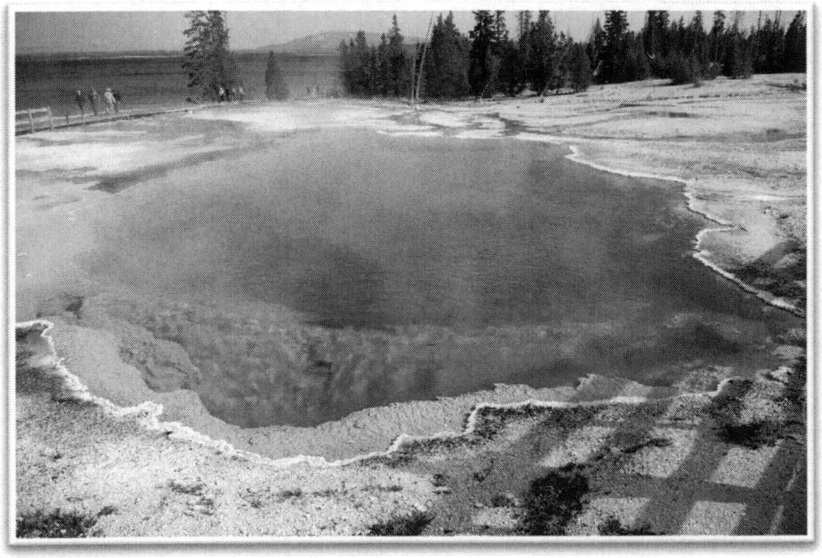

This can be as simple as putting on a warm pair of socks when your feet are cold, taking a sauna, or slipping into a hot spring or tub for a bath. By using external heat to elevate the body's internal temperature, enzymatic reactions are increased and the body has to do less work to reach the ideal 98.6° F.

"The reason that thermic applications and impressions are so powerful in arousing body functions lies in the fact that life activities are carried on only within a certain limited range of temperature."
— George Knapp Abbott

The higher your body temperature is, the greater the rate of chemical reactions will be. And an increased rate of chemical reactions means a higher metabolic rate. Again, body temperature is tied directly to your metabolic rate.

Water Transfers Temperature Better Than Air

Everybody knows that they will sweat if they sit in a sauna, but not too many people think about sweating while in a hot tub, hot spring, or hot bath. This is probably because there's no way to see beads of sweat on your soaking wet skin while fully submerged in water, but make no mistake about it, a lot of sweat is being released while bathing in hot water.

The warm or hot temperature of the water opens up the pores of the skin, which cleanses it by releasing any oils and dirt that happen to be in there.

Sweat is also released as a way to try to cool the body off when your temperature goes beyond 98.6° F. This happens much more efficiently in a hot tub than in a sauna to because the heat transfer through water is far more efficient than through air – "about 100 to 200 times faster," according to the US National Oceanic and Atmospheric Administration. This means that if you spent 20 minutes in a hot bath, you'd heat up quicker and release more sweat than you would spending equal time in a sauna.

And all this talk of saunas brings us to our next major benefit of elevating body temperature: detoxification.

Hot Water Detoxifies

Detoxification is the removal of anything toxic from the body that interferes with its proper function. There are many theories about detoxification and many products that claim they can help you detoxify, some of which work and some don't.

Many people turn to saunas as a form of detoxification. Nobody knows for sure where the first saunas were built, but the tradition is believed to originate somewhere in Northern Europe around 4000 years ago. And as it turns out, sitting in a wooden shack and dumping water on hot rocks heated by a wood burning stove is one of the best ways to remove chemicals from your body.

There have been a lot of naysayers in the past who've denied that a sauna could remove toxic chemicals from the body. Thankfully, in 2012, Canadian researchers Margaret Sears and her colleagues finally settled the score after publishing a large review of existing research on sweating and detoxification, which found...

- Arsenic dermal excretion was severalfold higher in arsenic-exposed individuals than in unexposed controls.
- Cadmium was more concentrated in sweat than in blood plasma.
- Mercury levels normalized with repeated saunas in a case report.

So, we know that sweating enables our bodies to release toxic chemicals from storage within our fat cells and eliminate them through our pores. This is undoubtedly one of the many beneficial things about hot water baths, and why historically they have been so medically important. In today's world, which contains infinitely more chemicals than even a hundred years ago, sweating and detoxification are of even greater importance for health maintenance or recovery.

There's one more benefit of warm baths over cold baths that I want to mention before concluding this chapter. It's the perfect segue into our next chapter on minerals.

Water Temperature and Mineral Content

On its way to the earth's surface, hot spring water passes through cracks in many layers of bedrock. Depending on the type of elements present in that rock, the resulting spring water can contain many different combinations and concentrations of mineral elements dissolved inside it.

Water temperature is an important factor in the concentration of minerals absorbed by that water: the hotter the temperature, the more minerals it can hold.

I don't want to get too nerdy technical on you, but it's important to explain a little more about this so you understand why that bath bomb in your bath eventually vanishes. Most solids tend to become more soluble in water with increasing temperature. This is true for sugar and salt, and it's true for other minerals as well.

Why is hot water a better solvent than cold water?

This has to do with the molecules inside hot water whirling around far more rapidly than when the water is cold. That increased energy results in increased collisions between the water molecules and the minerals, and voila! You have a solution which can dissolve more minerals at much more rapid rate.

Since hot water can hold a lot more minerals than cold water can, warm and hot springs are generally more highly saturated with minerals than cold springs.

But are minerals in the tub beneficial? And if so, which ones are the most beneficial? The impact of bathing in mineral-rich water on the body's metabolism will be the subject of our next chapter.

Minerals and the Ultimate Healing Bath

What did we discover about water temperature in this chapter that will help us create the most restorative bathing experience possible?

For the ultimate healing bath, alternating between cold and warm water baths might be ideal. But since this option might not be available to most people, prolonged hot water baths are an excellent option. Later in the book, we will expand upon this research and define exact temperature range for your bath water.

Conclusions

In the past, both hot water and cold water immersion have been used in balneotherapy.

In the short term, a quick dunk in cold water can powerfully stimulate heat production and metabolism in the body. However, anything more than a quick dip and you could be causing your body a great deal of stress. Glucose in your blood will be used up at an accelerated rate to warm up the body, and once that's all used up, stress hormones are released to begin breaking down and consuming your own tissues for energy. Since this would quickly lead to death, your body slows its metabolic rate as much as possible, which is the opposite of good health.

Your body temperature is tied directly to your metabolic rate. Normal body temperature is 98.6° F. If your temperature falls below that, your metabolic rate falls with it. Let it fall to 86° F and you'll literally have the same energy levels as a sloth. If you suffer from fatigue, and your body temperature is low, put on some warmer clothes or take a hot bath. Once your temperature reaches 98.6° F, or slightly higher, you'll feel noticeably more energized.

Hot water is an effective way to detoxify chemicals from your body. If you take saunas for detoxification, just remember that water transfers heat up to 200 times more effectively than through air. That's why a hot bath is far more effective at making your body sweat out toxic chemicals. Plus, in water, you're virtually weightless. How *cool* is that?

The final thing we covered in this chapter was the impact of water temperature on mineral solubility. The hotter your water, the more minerals you can dissolve inside it. The role of minerals and their health impact in balneotherapy will be the subject of our next chapter.

Key Points to Remember:

- Quick cold or ice bath immersions can powerfully stimulate your metabolism, by up to 280%.
- Prolonged bathing in cold water lowers body temperature, which induces stress and lowers your metabolic rate in order to preserve body tissues.

- Bathing in warm or hot water elevates the body temperature, which directly raises the metabolic rate.
- The thermal effects of warm water open up and cleanse the pores of the skin
- Bathing in water greater than 98.6° F promotes the safe release and elimination of toxic chemicals stored within fat cells.
- The ability of warm or hot water to store minerals is greater than that of cold water.

CHAPTER 4

MINERALS

Minerals are substances originally found within rock that can be used to make strong metal objects like copper pipes and iron skillets. They are also essential elements required by the human body to metabolize energy.

In nature, there are over 90 different soluble minerals, all of which the body needs. Very specific amounts of each of these minerals are required by the body – some are needed more than others – and maintaining a very specific ratio of one mineral relative to other minerals is also essential. In small amounts, minerals are required for your health, but in excess they become toxic heavy metals that can cause damage.

Right now, you're probably thinking how unbelievably complex the dance played by minerals inside the body seems to be – and how getting the right amounts of each mineral seems like an impossible task. Thankfully, this one has a happy ending. By the end of this chapter, any confusion about this will be resolved beautifully, so read on.

Minerals are intimately involved in the formation of bones and teeth, nerve function, they're an essential constituent in body fluids, and they are used to create enzymes which are essential for cellular energy production.

For example, the body requires the mineral magnesium and the vitamin B1 (thiamine) in order to create an essential metabolic enzyme called pyruvate dehydrogenase. Without magnesium or vitamin B1, this essential enzyme cannot be produced, which means your cells cannot use oxygen, which means less energy is produced by your cells, which means your metabolism slows. One more example is the mineral copper, which is essential for the creation of an essential enzyme called cytochrome c oxidase. Without copper, that enzyme cannot be produced, and metabolism fails. The same goes for a deficiency of any vitamin or minerals involved in the production of enzymes critical for cellular metabolism. Like a chain, when one link breaks, the entire chain malfunctions.

The bottom line is that minerals are essential for a high metabolism, and a deficiency in any one of them can slam on the metabolic brakes. Disease begins to manifest when the metabolism slows. The root cause of all chronic degenerative diseases is a dysfunctional metabolism.

Now that we've established that minerals are essential for a high metabolism, it's time to make things practical for us bath lovers and find out if the body can absorb and utilize the minerals contained in mineral-rich water. Other questions that we're going to answer in the remainder of this chapter include:

- Which minerals can be found in hot springs?
- Which minerals can be found in seas and oceans?
- Which combination of minerals added to a bath will give us the greatest metabolic benefit?

For this task, I've got a couple of important studies that will give us some answers.

Mineral Absorption Through Skin

Dr Rosemary Waring and her colleagues from the School of Biosciences at the University of Birmingham, UK conducted a study to find out if magnesium and sulfate dissolved in warm bath water could be absorbed through the skin. The study recruited 19 participants, ranging in age from 24-64 years. Each participant underwent one 12-minute bath with added Epsom salts (magnesium sulfate) every day for seven days. Blood samples and urine samples were taken following each bath and assessed. The study found that magnesium was elevated after the first bath in 16 of 19 subjects – and in the three subjects that didn't have elevated levels, there were elevated levels of magnesium in their urine, suggesting blood levels were optimal and the body was excreting the excess. In other words, **magnesium was absorbed through the skin of *all* subjects. Likewise, sulfate levels rose in the plasma of all subjects after bathing in Epsom salts.** And taking baths many days in a row resulted in a gradual accumulation of both magnesium and sulfate.

Yeehaw! Now we're making progress! We now know that minerals can be readily absorbed through the skin when dissolved in our bath water. But can the body use these minerals the same way they can if we consumed them in animal or plant foods? It might seem like the answer is an obvious yes, but there is actually some controversy surrounding the issue of inorganic minerals.

Here's the source of the drama: Minerals found in animal and plant foods are considered organic because they've been taken up into plants from the soil and processed organically, while crude minerals absorbed in baths or hot springs are considered inorganic because they're from rock and have never participated in life. Some sources have claimed that inorganic minerals "are perceived by the body as toxins" and that they "cannot bring life to cells," but evidence from thousands of years of balneotherapy use as well as modern scientific research both shatter this myth.

In 2017, scientists from Spain and France conducted a review of existing double-blind randomized clinical trials to determine if mineral elements and other chemical compounds played a therapeutic role in balneotherapy. Over 1100 patients with various diseases, including knee osteoarthritis, hand osteoarthritis, rheumatoid arthritis, low back pain and osteoporosis, were included in the review. Treatment groups in each of the studies were given mineral water baths and/or mud applications, and controls bathed in tap water and/or received "non-mineral" mud applications. **Mineral water or mud treatments "had better and longer improvements in pain, function, quality of life, clinical parameters, and others" than non-mineral mud and tap water bath treatments**, the study reports.

There we have it. Dissolved inorganic minerals in bath water can be absorbed and utilized by the body just like organic minerals can. I could show you literally dozens more studies showing that bathing in hot springs and salty seas provide benefit as well, but that will not be necessary. We now know beyond a shadow of a doubt that dissolved minerals inside baths are of therapeutic value.

The next order of business in this chapter is to determine which types of minerals can be found in hot springs and in oceans – and most importantly, which combinations of minerals will provide us the most benefit. Let's get to it.

Minerals Found in Hot Springs

Hot springs can contain any number of combinations of minerals and trace elements. It all depends on which elements were absorbed from the rock that the water interacted with on its way to the surface. Typically, in hot springs, you'll find calcium, sulfate, magnesium, iron, chloride, potassium, and zinc—to name a few.

In Japan, hot springs are used therapeutically for overcoming a variety of diseases. The Japanese name for hot spring is *Onsen*. Since Japan is a volcanic island, there are more naturally occurring hot springs than anywhere else in the world. In total, there are over 30,000 naturally occurring Onsens and 3,000 Onsen resorts in Japan. Compare that to the United States, which has around 1,600 naturally occurring hot springs and around 100 hot spring resorts.

Onsens are so important medically in Japanese culture that they actually created a law called the "Onsenhou" which, translated to English, means Hot Spring Law, and is used to determine which hot springs qualify as medical hot springs (Onsens) and which ones don't. In order to be considered an Onsen, a hot spring must be over a temperature of 25 degrees and must contain at least one of 19 different types of minerals.

By knowing the characteristics of each Onsen, you can help recharge your body with specific minerals. This is why hot spring resorts in Japan display the mineral spring qualities of each Onsen on the wall before entering.

After decades of research, leading Japanese Onsen researcher Dr. Yuko Agishi has shown that hot spring water, depending on its mineral composition, can help people recover from surgery and other conditions like joint and muscle pain (rheumatism), pain from nerve damage (neuralgia), high blood pressure (hypertension), and skin diseases.

Here are some of the different types of Onsens that exist in Japan:

1. Simple Onsen
2. Acidic Onsen
3. Alkaline Onsen
4. Sulfur Onsen
5. Sulfate Onsen
6. Sodium Chloride Onsen
7. Iron Onsen
8. Aluminum Onsen
9. Radium Onsen
10. Carbonated Onsen

Hot spring types similar to the ones listed above are probably found in many countries across the world. Ask my opinion on which one is best and I'll tell you that some are probably far better and far safer than others. I wouldn't dunk my toenail in some of them!

Simple Onsens

The simple hot spring is probably a good choice long term. They're generally fairly low in minerals so their primary benefit might be the temperature and the community between people that these baths create.

Acidic/Alkaline Onsens

The skin and bloodstream requires a very specific and delicate pH balance. Too much acidity or alkalinity in the bloodstream will cause a rise in stress hormones. So, bathing often in either an acid or alkaline hot spring without careful monitoring of your body's pH could easily damage your metabolism.

Sulfur/Sulfate Onsens

Our metabolisms require a steady supply of the mineral sulfur, which after calcium and phosphorus is the most abundant mineral in our bodies. People like MIT research scientist Stephanie Seneff have said that "sulfate deficiency is the most common nutritional deficiency" in our bodies. Because sulfur is inadequate in most people, sulfur and sulfate baths are probably some of the safer and more beneficial types of hot springs to use long term. But get ready for the smell of rotten eggs!

Sodium Chloride Onsens

Sodium and chloride (salt) are by far the most abundant mineral ions in the bloodstream. They are absolutely essential for life. The most common cause of death by endurance athletes is a condition called hyponatremia, which is low sodium concentration in the blood caused by drinking too much water. Sodium chloride hot springs and oceans are great choices for balneotherapy long term.

Iron/Aluminum Onsens

Iron and aluminum are required by the body, but only in very small amounts. In excess, these are both toxic heavy metals and powerful metabolic inhibitors. Bathing in hot springs with concentrated amounts of these minerals often can likely cause some serious problems.

Radium Onsens

Radium is a radioactive element, which means it emits ionizing radiation. There is no safe level of exposure to ionizing radiation. Anybody who has read my book *Cancer: The Metabolic Disease Unravelled* has seen the research on low-dose ionizing radiation themselves and will want to avoid bathing in radioactive hot springs like the plague. This is the Onsen type I was referring to above when I said I wouldn't dunk my toenail inside. From this point on, I will refer to radium Onsens as toenail Onsens.

Carbonated Onsens

Carbonated hot springs are like bathing in a bathtub full of soda pop. Well, minus the sugar, of course (unfortunately). Carbon dioxide plays a critical and very misunderstood role in the body's metabolism. You'll learn all about CO2s physiological importance in the next chapter. For now, I will mention that its role as an anti-oxidant, as a vasodilator, and its ability to shuttle oxygen into cells are among its long list of benefits.

That's it for my critique of all the different types of hot springs out there. I hope that has made you feel more confident about choosing which hot springs to visit and which to avoid.

This is where things get even more interesting. Instead of trying to pick and choose which kind of mineral soup we want to bathe in, why not bathe in water containing every essential mineral and trace element that the body needs?

All Rivers Lead to the Ocean

After droplets of rain fall from the clouds onto the surface of the earth, the rain then flows downhill, dissolving and accumulating minerals from the dirt and soil that it passes by along the way. Some of the rain water will end up in ponds or lakes where it will soak deep into the ground and recharge aquifers, and some runoff will make its way into small creeks and streams. Creeks and streams will flow until they combine to form a much larger river of flowing water.

As water in a large river flows downhill, it cuts into the earth – grinding up rocks, stirring up soil and incorporating a bounty of minerals in its flowing water. Mineralized river water continues to make its way downhill until ultimately it reaches its equilibrium and final destination – the ocean.

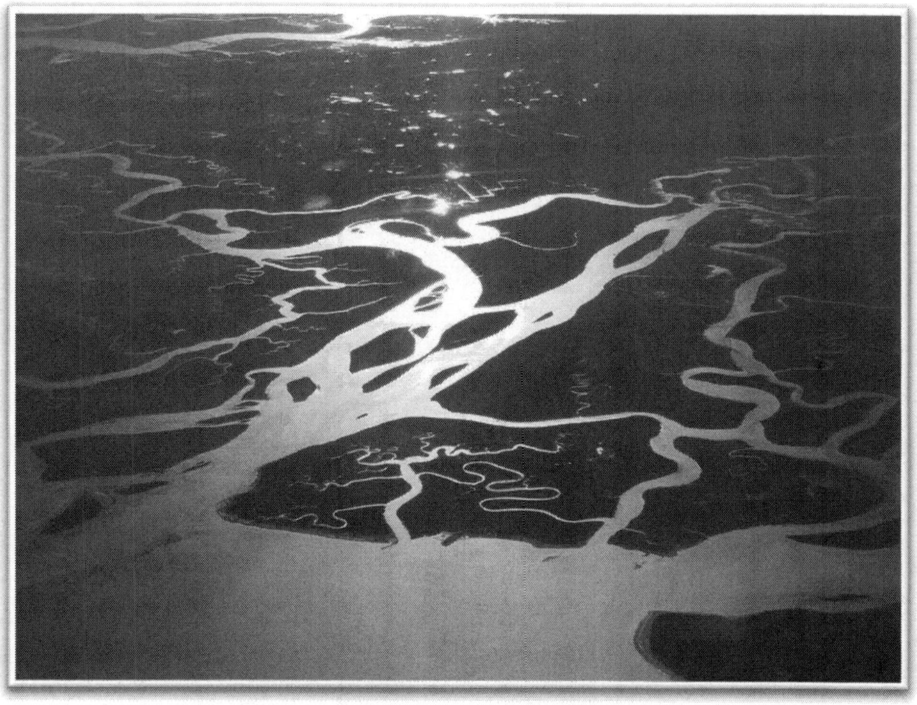

Image: A river delta is where rivers and the ocean meet.

That's right. All rivers eventually flow into the sea. This means that oceans receive a constant flow of water containing a constellation of every known mineral and trace element on earth.

Like mineral springs, seas and oceans are very important hubs for receiving the miraculous curative and cosmetic benefits of Balneotherapy. And you're about to find out why.

No Cancer in Sea Creatures

Dr. Maynard Murray was a 20th-century American biochemist, medical doctor, and research scientist who spent the majority of his life investigating the critical importance of minerals and trace elements to plant and animal life. After discussions with other scientists, Murray learned that cancer and cancerous tumors were rarely found in ocean life.

In order to find out for himself, Murray spent the next several years aboard fishing boats, where he dissected thousands of different species of sea creatures. Murray found no traces of cancer, heart disease or other degenerative diseases in any of the ocean life he dissected. One of the remarkable conclusions of his research was that biological aging does not occur in sea life. Murray knew there was something about the water itself that was responsible for the amazing well-being of ocean life, so he analyzed the mineral composition of sea water.

Dr. Murray discovered there were more than 90 water-soluble minerals and trace elements present within ocean water. Perhaps the most remarkable aspect of his discovery was that all of the minerals and trace elements contained within sea water were *in the exact proportions* required in the blood of all biological life. This point is so significant that it deserves an example to make it abundantly clear.

If you compare your typical mineral supplement found at your local health food store with ocean water, it would contain only a portion of the minerals that your body needs. Furthermore, the amount of each mineral contained in one capsule or tablet is simply the best guess of whoever created it as to what your body needs. Ocean water, on the other hand, contains every single mineral your body needs, and *in perfect balance*. This completely eliminates the need for guess work.

When an excessive amount of any element flows from rivers into the ocean, it precipitates out of the water and drops to the sea floor. This is how the perfect balance of elements is maintained in the ocean despite a constant flux of minerals delivered to it.

Could the lack of cancer that Dr. Murray discovered in sea life be explained by an ocean environment that's never deficient in the 90+ soluble elements found in nature?

Dr. Murray wondered if the alarming increase in chronic degenerative diseases among humans could be explained by the absence of minerals caused by eating foods grown in depleted soils.

Healthier Fruits and Vegetables Grown in Ocean Mineral Fertilizer

In order to test his theory, in 1938, Dr. Murray applied mineral salts from evaporated ocean water as fertilizer on vegetables, fruits and grains. His research demonstrated conclusively that plants fertilized with sea solids grew larger, faster, were vastly higher in nutrients, had longer shelf life and had greater resistance to disease than ones fertilized with conventional fertilizer. For example, a study on the growth of tomatoes was conducted in Northern Illinois. The experimental plot was fertilized with 2,200 pounds of dehydrated ocean minerals and the control plot was given conventional agriculture fertilizer. After the tomatoes had grown, experimenters discovered that tomatoes grown in the control plot had heavy blight from a fungus, and tomatoes grown in the soil that had been fertilized using ocean minerals were blight free and healthier looking (*Sea Energy Agriculture* p42). So, plants grown in soil fertilized using ocean minerals are much healthier, but what about the animals (and people) that eat them?

No Tumors in Rats Fed Ocean Mineral-Fertilized Chow

A number of experiments were then sanctioned by Dr. Murray to test the impact of feeding various animals food grown in soil fertilized with ocean minerals. In one study, 50 rats were divided into two groups, and one group was fed chow grown in conventionally fertilized soils, and the other was fed chow grown in soil fertilized with ocean minerals. While consuming these two diets, both groups of rats were injected with a type of cancerous tissue called Jensen Carcino-Sarcoma to determine if the ocean mineral diet would offer any protection from the disease. **21 days later, all of the rats fed the control diet had died.** And of the rats given the ocean mineral fertilized chow, nine died within 40 days, and sixteen survived a full 150 days before they were sacrificed for examination. When scientists autopsied the experimental rats, they found no cancerous tumors.

If you're like me, you're horrified by the fact that scientists would do such things to rats and other creatures in the name of science. I'm definitely against these types of experiments, however, this particular experiment has already been done, so there's no sense in wasting our energy over it. Instead, let's honor the rats by learning and applying to our lives the lessons that the experiment taught us. When my mom died of cancer, I used the pain inside to motivate me to research and write two monumental books on cancer – similarly, bettering ourselves with information from the rat study is the greatest honor we can give to those rats.

Given the fact that animals fed plants grown in ocean mineral fertilizer had greater resistance to disease, among many other health benefits that suggest high metabolic rates, and given what we know about the importance of minerals in the production of enzymes that power metabolic energy production within every cell, it is highly likely that humans too have much to gain from eating plants grown in ocean mineral fertilizer – and animals that were fed plants grown in ocean mineral fertilizer. It is also highly likely that humans can gain these same benefits from bathing in ocean water, or in baths containing dehydrated ocean mineral solids.

Maynard Murray's Main Message

Dr. Maynard Murray has taught us that the ocean is the perfect mineral source with which to supercharge our bath water. Ocean minerals are the most complete source of minerals that will award bathers the greatest possible benefit.

For all you gardeners out there who are now eager to get your hands on some ocean mineral fertilizer for your victory gardens, they can be found at seaagri.com. (These, of course, can also be used in the bath tub). I'm not affiliated with them, but they make a fantastic product. Another option for gardeners is to ask your local plant nursery for compost made from algae or other sea plants.

Quick question: which body of water is 9.6 times more salty than the ocean and so dense in minerals that when you enter it your body will float like a cork?

The Dead Sea Gives Life

The Dead Sea is a salt lake located directly on the border between Jordan (to the East) and Israel (to the West). Its soothing mineral waters have a rich history of therapeutic use by locals and tourists alike dating back thousands of years.

At almost 1500 feet below sea level, the salty shores of the Dead Sea are the lowest land elevation on earth. In biblical Christianity, Jesus was baptized in the Jordan River, which is the main river supplying water to the Dead Sea.

If you haven't guessed, the Dead Sea was given its name because its waters are too salty to support aquatic fish or other creatures. But the people who bathe in it know that the Dead Sea gives life.

While seawater in the world's oceans has an average salinity of 35g/L, the salinity of Dead Sea water is a whopping 348g/L. That's nearly 10x saltier!

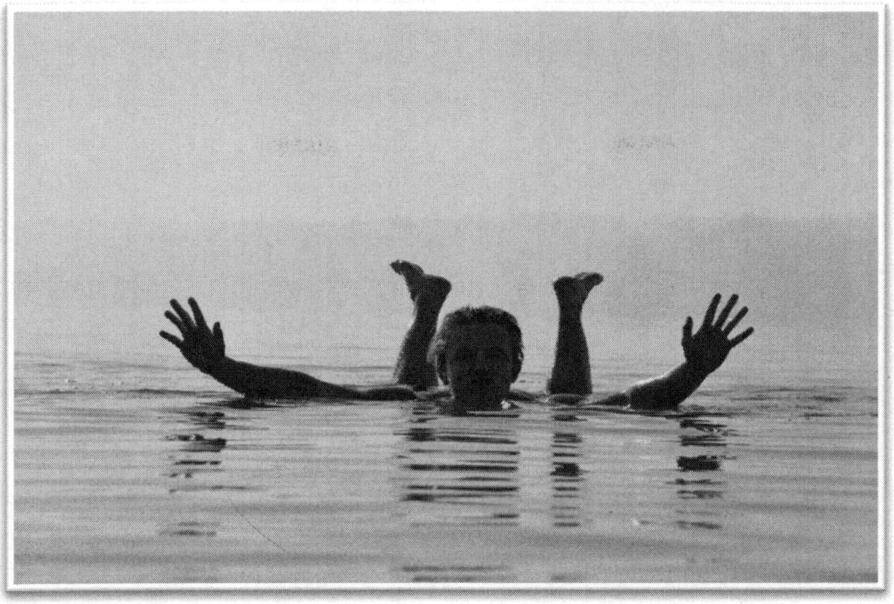

Image: Floating is easy on the Dead Sea

The climate surrounding the Dead Sea is a hot and dry desert, with average air temperatures in summer of about 35 degrees Celsius and about 21 degrees Celsius in winter.

In 2019, Israel welcomed 4.55 million visitors from all over the world to bathe in the Dead Sea brine. Today, there are countless beauty products on the market which include Dead Sea minerals.

One of the mysteries of the Dead Sea is the occasional presence of large blocks of asphalt floating on its surface. Even scientists aren't certain where the asphalt originates, but what we do know is they've been here since antiquity.

The two most plausible theories I've encountered come from a study in 1979 by scientists Ora Amit and Amos Bein, who wrote, "The oils, which are thought to be the precursors of the asphalts, have either been flushed into the Dead Sea depression from the surrounding elevated areas or have seeped upwards from deep local accumulations in the graben [earth's crust]."

Either way, like the unwrapped chocolate bar floating in the public pool like a turd in the 1980s film *Caddyshack*, hunks of asphalt are floating on the surface of the Dead Sea right now. Fascinatingly, this asphalt was an important item of trade in ancient times, especially for Egyptians who used it in the mummification process.

192 patients with psoriasis who had been sent to the Dead Sea, Israel for a four-week treatment of sun exposure and bathing were studied by Danish scientists from Bispebjerg Hospital, Copenhagen in 1996. After four weeks of therapy, 73% of the patients were completely (or almost completely) healed, and 20% of the 163 patients were significantly improved. The benefits lasted one to three months.

The Dead Sea might be the utmost balneotherapy experience in the entire world. It's interesting to note that the mineral content of the Dead Sea is actually very different from ocean water, and it also varies with the changing seasonal temperatures of the water.

While ocean water contains 85% sodium chloride and 15% other minerals and trace elements, Dead Sea water contains an entirely different mineral profile. The Dead Sea is more abundant in chloride, magnesium, sodium, calcium, potassium and bromide that are the world's oceans. The presence of sodium and high concentration of the alkaline minerals magnesium, calcium and potassium are all very beneficial. But ultimately, the Dead Sea is primarily a magnesium chloride lake.

Magnesium is an extremely important mineral in which about 70% of American's are deficient. When we're deficient in magnesium, over 300 enzymes in our body are unable to function properly. The magnesium in the Dead Sea is probably one of the main reasons for the incredible rejuvenation people receive while bathing in it.

"Magnesium is nothing short of a miracle mineral in its healing effect on a wide range of diseases as well as in its ability to rejuvenate the ageing body. We know that it is essential for many enzyme reactions, especially in regard to cellular energy production, for the health of the brain and nervous system and also for healthy teeth and bones. However, it may come as a surprise that in the form of magnesium chloride it is also an impressive infection fighter."

— Walter Last

One of the major downsides of Dead Sea water from a therapeutic perspective, relative to ocean water, is its low concentrations of sulfate, bicarbonate and all the other minerals and trace elements that ocean water contains. This limitation, of course, can be easily overcome when bathing in a bath tub, which we will talk about later.

Concentration of Minerals in Dead Sea vs. Ocean water

Mineral Contents	Dead Sea	Ocean
Sodium chloride	31%	85%
Calcium chloride	14%	1%
Potassium chloride	4%	1%
Magnesium chloride	51%	4%
90+ other minerals and trace elements	X	✓

Although the waters of the Dead Sea cannot currently support aquatic or plant life, and many people share great concern about its rapidly receding water level, biblical prophecy in Ezekiel 47:8-9 states that at some point in the future the sea will "be healed and made fresh" and capable of supporting aquatic life once more.

Conclusions

Mineral elements are essential ingredients for the lives of humans, animals, and all biological life on earth. The human body requires specific amounts of each mineral in precise balance with all other minerals for a high metabolic rate.

In a perfect world, all minerals would be obtained from food, but modern agriculture – which is essentially like mining the minerals from the land – has depleted soils significantly since it began. As a result, most modern diets are inadequate to provide the minerals (not to mention other nutrients) required by the body.

Thankfully, the move towards regenerative farming – that is, farming in a way that produces food while remineralizing and regenerating the soil and improving the environment in a myriad of ways – is on the rise. Supporting a local regenerative farmer and consuming their food can go a long way in improving the body's mineral intake as well as halting the destructive practices of modern agriculture and reversing the ecological damage it has caused.

But a much more rapid way for us to nourish our bodies with minerals in perfect balance is to bathe in warm, ocean mineral-rich water. We've demonstrated that dissolved "inorganic" mineral ions are efficiently absorbed through the skin during balneotherapy, and are as readily used as "organic" minerals are once inside the body.

We've learned that hot springs have their advantages and disadvantages. The diversity of mineral contents from one hot spring to the next can either be a blessing or a curse. Generally, hot springs will likely contain a bounty of different minerals and will be a great choice for your balneotherapy sessions, but some hot springs, for example, ones containing large amounts of radioactive mineral ions, known as *toenail Onsens*, could potentially cause harm.

In search of the ultimate revitalizing bath water, ocean waters are of great interest because they contain over 90 minerals and trace elements, in *perfect balance* as required by human blood serum and probably by all biological life. From the viewpoint of its dissolved mineral content, no water found in the natural world could be more ideal for balneotherapy than ocean water.

One of the saltiest bodies of water in the world, which people eager to receive its gifts have flocked to for literally thousands of years, is the Dead Sea. Bathing in the warm magnesium chloride waters of the Dead Sea will give patients a potent dose of important alkaline minerals, while simultaneously providing lots of red, near-infrared and UV phototherapy from the sun. The Dead Sea can be considered a fast lane to recovery for the nearly 50% of the world's population who are deficient in vitamin D and the 70% who are deficient in magnesium.

Minerals and the Ultimate Healing Bath

What did we discover about minerals that we can use to create the ultimate therapeutic bathing experience for ourselves at home?

For the ultimate bath recipe, the ideal mineral source to add that's the most complete is dehydrated ocean minerals. Additionally, adding Dead Sea salts or Epsom salts (magnesium sulfate) will make it better.

Add 1-2 lbs. of ocean minerals to your bath and 1-2 lbs. of Dead Sea salts (or Epsom salts) to create the ultimate mineral profile in your baths at home.

Key Points to Remember

- Minerals are required by the body for a number of functions, including to power metabolism within cells.
- Minerals dissolved in water are readily absorbed through the skin during a bath.
- Baths containing minerals are more beneficial for health than non-mineral baths.

- Hot springs can contain a number of different minerals depending on the minerals contained within the rock the water interacted with on its way to the Earth's surface.
- Over 90 water-soluble minerals and trace elements exist within ocean water; all of which are essential for human health.
- The minerals contained within ocean water are *in the exact proportions* required by the blood serum of humans, animals and other biological life.
- Sea creatures almost never get cancerous tumors, heart disease, or other degenerative diseases.
- Biological aging does not occur in ocean life.
- Plants fertilized with sea solids grew larger, faster, were vastly higher in nutrients, had longer shelf life, and had greater resistance to disease.
- Animals fed diets containing food grown in soils fertilized using ocean minerals have greater disease resistance and superior overall health.
- The waters of the Dead Sea, which are almost 10x as salty as ocean water, have been used for thousands of years for recovery.
- The Dead Sea is primary a magnesium chloride lake; and around 70% of people are deficient in magnesium.
- Add 1-2 lbs. of ocean minerals to your bath and 1-2 lbs. of Dead Sea salts (or Epsom salts) to create the ultimate mineral profile in your baths at home.

CHAPTER 5

CARBONATION

Ever bathed in a tub of champagne? Me neither. But this is how some people have described the experience of bathing in a carbon dioxide bath.

Here's a breakdown of the many different sections in this chapter:

- History of carbon dioxide baths
- Carbon dioxide effects on metabolism
- Replicating the Nauheim bath at home
- Five modern carbon dioxide therapies

History of Carbon Dioxide Baths

The carbon dioxide bath originated in the German town of Nauheim, which is known for its natural carbonated hot springs. And yes, it is exactly what it sounds like – bathing in water containing tiny bubbles of carbon dioxide.

When you first slip into a carbon dioxide bath, you'll notice the water is a bit cooler than you may have expected – between 86-95° F. Once fully immersed, tiny bubbles of carbon dioxide gas immediately begin to accumulate on the skin of your entire body. The micro bubbles initially create a cooling sensation on the skin, but the carbon dioxide quickly goes to work dilating your blood vessels and increasing blood flow to your skin, which replaces the feeling of cold with a soothing warmth.

There are a number of other names for the carbon dioxide bath, including effervescent bath, carbonic acid bath, and Nauheim bath, after its city of origin.

"The Nauheim bath became famous for the treatment of heart disease and was considered by some as the panacea for all cardiac ailments," wrote Naturopath Sussanna Czeranko in an article titled *The History of Carbonated Water and Nauheim Baths.* Traditionally, Nauheim baths were a foundational therapy for every diseases and conditions of all kinds. The standard protocol for Nauheim baths in Nauheim consisted of a series of 18 to 24 baths.

Hot springs become naturally carbonated as a result of deep underground mineral waters filtering through volcanic soils containing carbon dioxide, according to scientists Gabriela Dogaru and Alexandru Radulescu in a paper published in *Balneo Research Journal* in 2015. The result is an incredibly refreshing and mind-blowingly therapeutic bathing experience.

One of the most unique carbonated bathing experiences can be found at a traditional Japanese Inn, located in the heart of the Nagayu Onsen hot springs district, called Daimaru Ryokan. This inn contains a carbonated spring with CO2 concentrations so high that you can literally see the fizzing water. And while bathing in it, your entire body will be covered in silver bubbles.

Carbonated hot springs exist all over the world, and are abundant in places like Europe and Japan, but in other places, like North America, they are few and far between. Saratoga, New York, California, and Idaho are among the few places in the United States which have naturally occurring carbonated springs. The carbonated hot springs in Soda Springs, Idaho are an interesting story that I'll briefly talk about now.

Soda Springs, Idaho is home to thousands of naturally carbonated springs. In 1937, an attempt was made to create a natural hot springs swimming pool by drilling down near the springs, but they got the surprise of a lifetime: a geyser erupted and began shooting a thick stream of carbonated spring water 100 feet into the air.

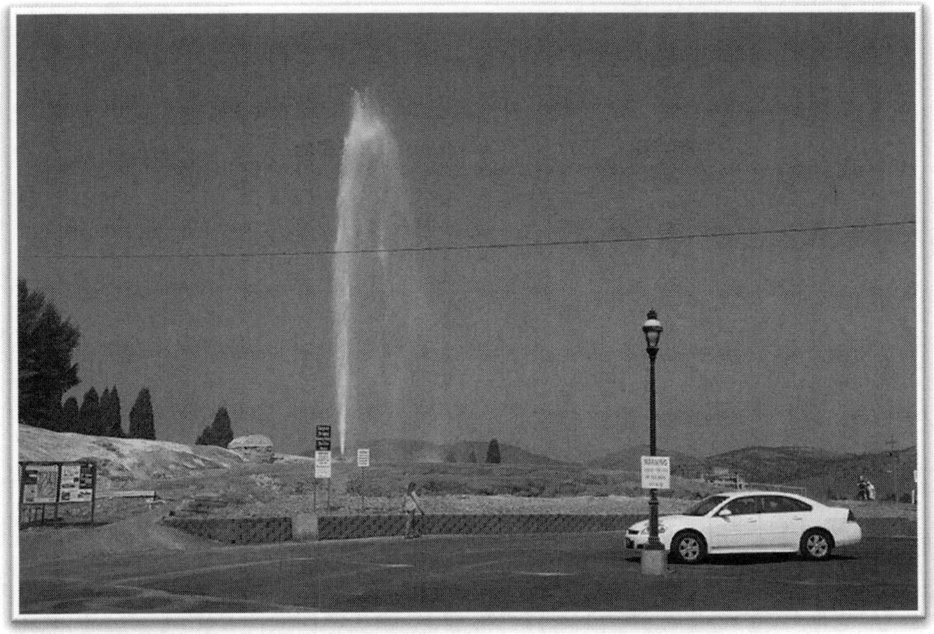

Image: The Soda Springs geyser erupting in Idaho.

Since then, the famous geyser has been capped and erupts on a timer once every hour. A park and visitor's center has been built at the site. Oh, and in case you were wondering, even though the attempt to make a swimming pool failed and resulted in a geyser, there are plenty of hot springs in Soda Springs, Idaho for you to visit.

Anyway, due to the rarity of carbonated hot springs in America – and also due to the fact that few people could afford to travel to Europe – American doctors came up with a solution that would allow patients who don't live near a carbonated mineral spring to still benefit from one: The "Artificial" or simulated Nauheim bath – designed to replicate spring water qualities of the carbonated bath springs in Nauheim, Germany – was born.

It was the year 1835 when balneotherapy clinics offering effervescent carbonic acid baths began to flourish in North America. Doctors created their own formulations of ingredients to add to baths that they believed most accurately simulated a Nauheim bath and its therapeutic effects.

You may remember me writing about Dr. John Harvey Kellogg in my book *Red Light Therapy: Miracle Medicine* where I discussed his use of ultraviolet phototherapy in his medical practices. Well, the same man who brought you your corn flakes and other products was also the superintendent in charge of caring for patients with carbon dioxide-based balneotherapy at the Battle Creek Sanitarium, in Michigan, USA.

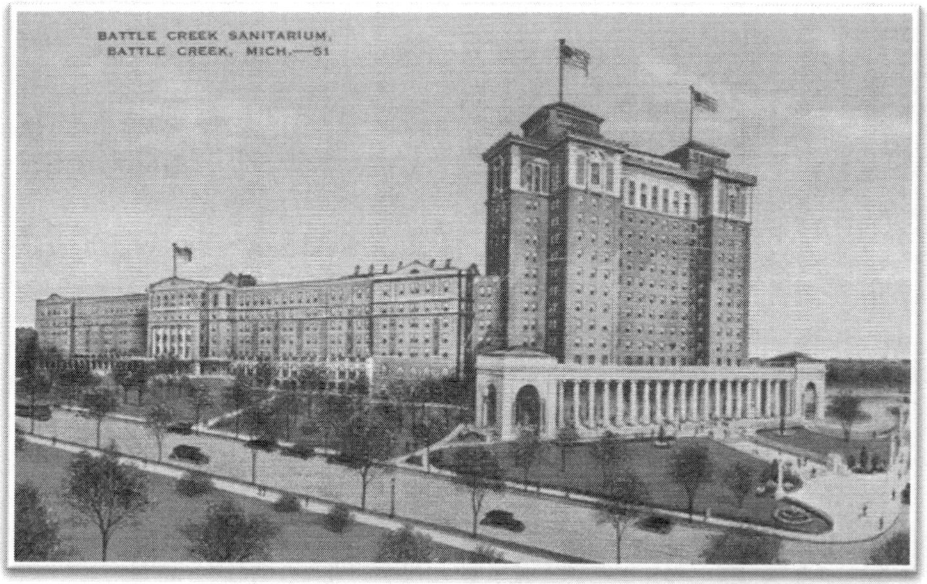

Image: The Battle Creek Sanitarium headed by Dr. John Harvey Kellogg in Battle Creek, Michigan

By the 1850s, heaps of spa villages emerged across 20 states, including over 2,000 hot- and cold-spring resorts. Not only were these clinics all over the US and in other western countries, but the name of these establishments says it all: "Water Cure."

In addition to carbonated mineral baths, many of the water therapy centers also emphasized diet and exercise to their patrons, who were pampered in large buildings with lavish facilities – under the supervision of fully trained medical practitioners and staff – often for weeks at a time.

Most people will be surprised to hear that prior to the 1940s, when Western medicine was reduced to the use of knives and synthetic drugs, carbon dioxide baths (and simulated carbon dioxide baths) were a primary therapy for many conditions. In fact, the foundation of Western medicine for literally thousands of years has been bathing in water in one form or another.

In the United States, diseases traditionally treated with simulated carbon dioxide baths include:

- Arteriosclerosis
- Hypertension
- Angina
- Chronic Nephritis
- Cardiac weakness
- Rheumatism

For about one hundred years, masses of people benefitted from effervescent carbonic acid baths used for insomnia, anemia, loss of appetite, impotence, old age, circulatory problems, hemorrhoids, irregular menstruation, heart disease, rheumatism, gout, and skin diseases. According to some of the most distinguished doctors of the day, water was curative for everything from anxiety to cancer.

"The Nauheim, or carbon dioxide bath, continues to be used in several European countries as part of a flourishing network of medical balneotherapy clinics. Here in North America, this remarkable modality has simply vanished into thin air," writes Czeranko.

Carbon Dioxide Effects on Metabolism

"Over the oxygen supply of the body carbon dioxide spreads its protecting wings."

– Friedrich Miescher, Swiss physiologist, 1885

With the remarkable ability of Balneotherapy to address many ailments, you might be wondering how it all works.

You'll recall from our chapter on metabolism that a high metabolism is the definition of health, and that the presence of unwanted symptoms or diseases in the body is indicative of metabolic dysfunction. The question is: How does CO2 affect cellular metabolism?

When students of biology or medicine at University are taught about cellular metabolism, they learn about the complex process called oxidative phosphorylation, which basically means a set of chemical reactions that occur within the mitochondria of cells to essentially oxidize molecules of glucose. One of the things they are taught has resulted in an absolute misunderstanding of carbon dioxide. The American College of Cardiology has it written on their website: "Carbon dioxide (CO2) is a gaseous waste product from metabolism." But carbon dioxide plays such an essential role in metabolism that this couldn't be farther from the truth. I will do my best to keep this simple, and few things are more worthwhile understanding, so read on.

CO2 is so central to a healthy metabolism that – rather than a waste product – scientist Kyle Mamounis has called carbon dioxide *The Product* of cellular metabolism.

More than 90% of the carbon dioxide in your blood stream exists in the form of bicarbonate (HC03). The remainder of the CO2 is either dissolved carbon dioxide gas (CO2) or carbonic acid (H2CO3).

Carbon dioxide has a myriad of beneficial effects in the body, including its role as a powerful anti-oxidant and anti-inflammatory. But the two most important effects of carbon dioxide exhibit on the body include vasodilation and its role in *The Bohr Effect.* We will briefly go over these now.

CO2: The Body's Primary Vasodilator

In the bloodstream, one of carbon dioxide's primary roles is to dilate blood vessels. This allows for increased blood circulation throughout the entire body, which is one of the main reasons why CO2 baths are so effective at reducing high blood pressure and other cardiac ailments.

"Carbonated water baths increase arteriolar blood flow in the skin, the vasodilator effect being directly proportional to the carbon dioxide concentration in the mineral bath."

— Scientists Gabriela Dogaru and Alexandru Radulescu

Even bathing just one limb inside carbonated water can result in significant improvements in blood flow to that area. A study published in the *European Journal of Applied Physiology* in 2002 reported that "Cutaneous blood flow in the immersed skin (right forearm) was significantly increased during CO2 bathing compared with that during fresh-water bathing."

In 1997, German researchers from the University of Freiburg compared the effects of soaking the lower legs of people in either fresh water or in carbon dioxide enriched water (1200mg CO2 per kg water). While legs immersed in fresh water were found to have no increase in circulation and little increase in oxygen use, researchers discovered that circulation in legs immersed in carbon dioxide enriched water was enhanced by 300% and oxygen pressure within tissues was increased by 10%.

These remarkable findings are worth repeating: CO2 baths (at 1200mg CO2/kg) resulted in 300% better blood circulation and 10% increased oxygen use.

Ultimately, increased blood flow in the body means increased delivery of oxygen and other nutrients to all your cells and tissues as well as better removal of dead cellular debris and other wastes. This increased efficiency means a more robust metabolism.

CO2 & The Bohr Effect

In my book, *Cancer: The Metabolic Disease Unravelled,* I explained the Bohr Effect in this way:

> *"...oxygen is transported through the bloodstream bound to red blood cells (hemoglobin), and the primary trigger for the release of oxygen from hemoglobin (the Bohr effect) is carbon dioxide. In other words, without CO2, oxygen cannot get into cells where it is needed."*

To help this critical information soak in, I'll break it down for you again in a slightly different way: Without carbon dioxide, your cells can't use oxygen. And without oxygen, mitochondrial metabolism will fail. The metabolic dysfunction that results can be found in all chronic degenerative diseases.

Lack of Oxygen = The Root Cause of Disease

In 1976, a remarkable statement was made by the author of one of the most widely used medical textbooks in the world, *The Textbook of Medical Physiology*:

"All chronic pain, suffering and diseases are caused from a lack of oxygen at the cell level."

-Dr. Arthur C. Guyton

By increasing carbon dioxide in the body therapeutically, the delivery and use of oxygen inside all cells of the body is increased – correcting what Dr. Guyton has identified as *the root cause* of all pain, suffering and disease.

This extraordinary claim of course requires extraordinary proof. So rather than expecting you to believe Dr. Guyton, I'll tell you briefly about the fascinating life's work of the elite Russian scientist Dr. Konstantin Buteyko and how it relates.

The Extraordinary Discovery of Dr. Buteyko

Dr. Konstantin Buteyko was an elite scientist engaged in research for the Russian military, space, and sports programs in the early 20th century. He had the most state-of-the-art equipment and facilities in the world at his disposal, which he used to try and find an answer to the question that he was most passionate about answering: *What are the physiological and biochemical differences between a person who is healthy and a person with disease?*

After collecting data from hundreds of different patients over the course of many years, Buteyko made what was undoubtedly the most revolutionary discovery in the history of medicine: **all people suffering from chronic diseases are deficient in carbon dioxide.**

Dr. Buteyko found that people who had optimal levels of carbon dioxide never suffered from any chronic diseases – and the greater the deficiency of carbon dioxide a person had, the worse their overall level of health. For the record, the medical norm of carbon dioxide concentration in the human body is around 5% (or 35-37mm Hg).

"The presence of carbon dioxide is an indicator of proper mitochondrial respiratory functioning."

— Ray Peat, PhD

And I'm going to lay down some more evidence in favor of Guyton's statement, from my book *Cancer: The Metabolic Disease Unravelled.*

Scientific experiments have determined that people with a wide variety of diseases are deficient in carbon dioxide, including heart disease, diabetes, asthma, COPD, sleep apnea, cystic fibrosis, bipolar disorder, panic disorder, epilepsy, and cancer.

To recap, lack of oxygen is the root cause of all pain, suffering and disease, and carbon dioxide is the linchpin that determines whether or not your body can use oxygen. Dr. Buteyko's discovery validated Dr. Guyton's statement by revealing that there was a lack of carbon dioxide inside all people with illness and disease.

Enough of this technical talk of metabolism for now! Let's make this practical and I'll show you how to charge water with carbon dioxide inside your own bath tub.

Replicating the Nauheim bath at home

So you want to create a carbon dioxide bath for yourself at home? There are two known ways you can do this:

1. **Using Carbonated Minerals:** By adding a combination of ingredients to your bath, a reaction will take place that produces bubbles of carbon dioxide gas. Think *bath bombs.*

2. **Using Compressed Carbon Dioxide Gas:** By infusing carbon dioxide gas directly into the water using a cylinder of compressed CO2.

Below we will go over both of these methods in depth so you can understand everything you need to know to properly administer these therapies to yourself at home.

1. Using Carbonated Minerals

To produce the carbon dioxide gas in the bath, it is necessary that an acid come in contact with an alkaline carbonate, which liberates the carbon dioxide.

By adding baking soda (sodium bicarbonate) powder to your bath, you are essentially adding salt bound to carbon dioxide. By adding some kind of acid along with it, the bicarbonate ions will be converted into carbonic acid which is rapidly absorbed by the body. These are the two primary ingredients in a bath bomb. In the case of a bath bomb, sodium bicarbonate reacts usually with citric acid to create tiny bubbles of carbon dioxide.

The formulation developed and used by Dr. Kellogg's to recreate the waters of Nauheim inside baths at the Battle Creek Sanitarium included:

- Sodium carbonate: 1½ lb
- Sodium bicarbonate (baking soda): ½ lb
- Calcium chloride: 3 lb
- Sodium chloride: 2 lb
- Sodium bisulphate: 1 lb

In this formulation, the baking soda was converted into carbon dioxide (which is called carbonic acid when dissolved in water) by the addition of the acid sodium bisulphate.

2. Using Compressed Carbon Dioxide Gas

American physician Dr. Simon Baruch studied the differences between naturally carbonated spring water and artificially carbonated water used in balneotherapy. One of Dr. Baruch's key discoveries was that adding minerals to a carbon dioxide bath increased CO2 absorption and prevented the escape of CO2 from the water.

On a practical level, this means that if you choose to create your carbon dioxide baths using a cylinder of compressed CO2 gas, you should also add minerals to the bath; they will allow both the water and your body to absorb more CO2.

In his 1919 book *Rational Therapy*, Otto Lerch describes one such formula, which included sodium chloride and calcium chloride added to a bath fortified also with carbon dioxide gas from a compressed air tank.

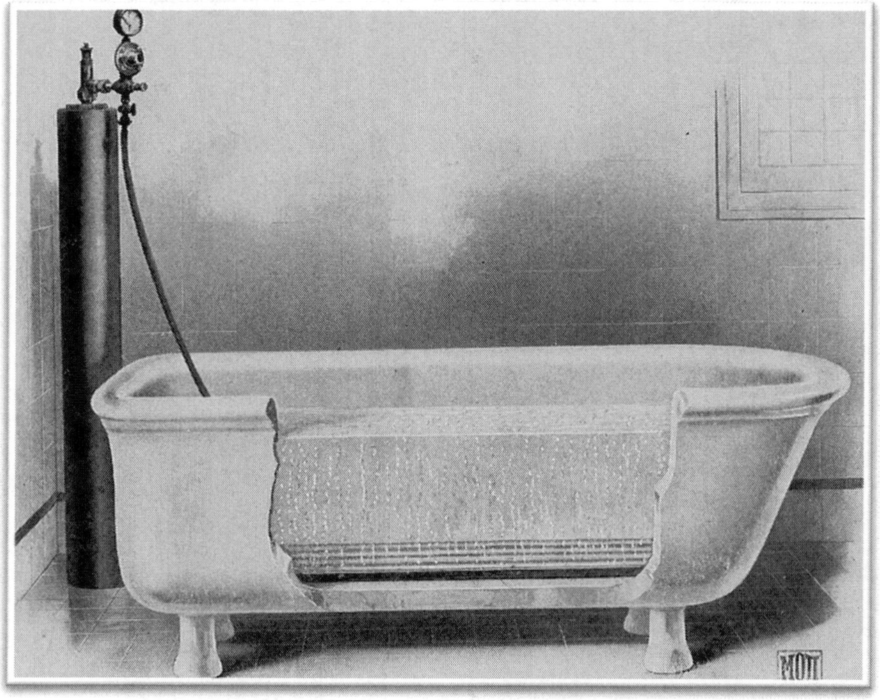

Image: A bath containing dissolved sodium chloride and calcium chloride and carbonated using gas from a compressed cylinder. From the book *Rational Therapy* (1919).

Lerch continues, "The imported Nauheim Salt, consisting principally of Sodium Chloride and Calcium Chloride may be added to the bath to increase its stimulating effects. It is important that the Carbon dioxide surrounds the patient with fine gas pearls that adhere to the skin. Only when that is the case, is the bath effective. The bath is generally commenced with a temperature of 90° F and a duration of from seven to ten minutes. As the patient improves, the temperature is lowered and the time prolonged. The same course is generally pursued with the composition of the bath. A smaller quantity is first used to prepare it, and this is gradually increased during the course of the treatment. The patient has an agreeable prickling sensation when in the bath, is less sensitive to lower temperatures and reacts promptly, the skin reddens after a few-minutes of exposure."

CO_2 Baths Enhance Athletic Performance

Some interesting research has been done on the impact of carbonated baths on athletic performance. Japanese scientists from the National Institute of Fitness and Sports in Kanoya, Japan conducted a study in 1998 that had swimmers warm up by bathing in an artificially carbonated bath before swimming. The water temperature was 96° F, the CO_2 concentration in the water was 300ppm, and the bath lasted 20 minutes. The scientists observed that the warm-up effects of a carbonated bath in swimmers significantly increased important blood components like red and white blood cells during the swim and significantly reduced changes in heart rate and blood lactic acid content after the swim. In other words, swimmers that took carbonated baths as a warmup before swimming had "better performance during swimming and less accumulation of fatigue-related metabolites after swimming."

The Importance of Water Temperature

Something to keep in mind is the importance of maintaining water temperature within a specific range when pouring a carbon dioxide bath. A simple thermometer should be used to reach the desired temperature. You'll recall the water temperature Lerch recommended in his writings to use in carbonated baths was 90° F.

The reason for the lower temperature is that while most minerals and other solids, including sugar and salt, become increasing soluble with increasing temperature, the opposite is true for a gas. As temperature increases, less carbon dioxide gas is able to dissolve in the water. The result of water too warm is that molecules of CO_2 gas will break free from the liquid and into the air where they cannot be absorbed through the skin. This is why carbonated drinks quickly "go flat" when left at room temperature or when heated.

Doctors at hydrotherapy facilities carefully monitored water temperature in carbonated baths for their patients, maintaining a temperature ranging between 86-95° F – and you should, too.

5 Modern Carbon Dioxide Therapies

There are a number of other very interesting and effective ways to administer carbon dioxide therapy that are worth noting. Here are five examples that I'll go over:

1. Dry Carbon Dioxide Baths
2. Carboxytherapy
3. Carboxytherapy Gel
4. Carbon Dioxide Face Baths
5. Drinking Carbonated Water

If you're interested in CO2 Therapy, I've created a list of high-quality products with discount codes on the following page:
https://www.endalldisease.com/store/#CARBON_DIOXIDE_THERAPY

1. Dry Carbon Dioxide Baths

The first type of CO2 therapy I'm going to introduce to you is the *dry* carbon dioxide bath. Unlike a wet carbon dioxide bath, which is taken inside a tub of water, a dry carbon dioxide bath involves entering a large bag or bodysuit up to your neck. Once sealed inside, carbon dioxide is pumped into the bag or suit from a compressed cylinder. The patient remains inside the bag until all of the CO2 is absorbed through the skin.

Carbon dioxide dry baths are good for skin conditions and every disease that benefits from elevating the body's metabolic rate. According to Naturopath Sussanna Czeranko, "Just ten to 15 treatments of the dry carbon dioxide baths are sufficient in restoring cellulite tissue to a firm and smooth appearance." She says a typical protocol consists of two to three baths per week.

Studies have also shown CO2 dry baths have a dramatic effect on the recovery of heart attack patients. The following is an excerpt from a Russian study published in 1989:

"A group of 75 patients with a history of myocardial infarction and repeated myocardial infarction were subjected to treatment involving dry carbon dioxide baths. Its results demonstrated normalization of IHD manifestations, such as coronary and heart failure, functional state of the cardiovascular system, its reserve potentialities and adaptation to physical effort. **Under the influence of a course treatment with dry carbon dioxide baths, hemodynamic parameters of cardiac output (cardiac and stroke volume) underwent favourable changes, rhythm slowed down, diastole became longer and systolic and diastolic arterial pressure decreased.**"

These full-body dry CO2 baths are offered in many European spas. According to one study, the "optimal concentration range [is] between 1000 and 1400 mg/L."

Commercially manufactured, air-tight body suits designed to administer dry CO2 baths can also be purchased for at-home use. One such company is *Carbogenetics,* owned by a friend of mine who I've teamed up with in selling his fantastic products. One of his inventions is a *CO2 dry bath bodysuit device*, and the other is his own unique innovation: a *CO2 infrared sauna*, both of which are available on the Endalldisease store. The advantage of the CO2 sauna is that the sweat released from your skin while using it will actually increase the absorption rate of carbon dioxide through your skin.

2. Carboxytherapy

Carboxytherapy is a non-invasive cosmetic procedure popular today for a number of conditions like obesity, cellulite, and stretch marks. Carboxytherapy involves the use of expensive equipment to inject carbon dioxide gas directly under the skin using a needle.

Carbon dioxide can accelerate wound repair. In 2010, a Greek study tested the effects of carboxytherapy injections on 70 patients affected by chronic ulcers. The study reports that "In the group that underwent subcutaneous treatment with CO(2) therapy, the results highlighted a significant increase in tissue oxygenation values, which was confirmed by greater progress of the lesions in terms of both healing and reduction of the injured area."

Carboxytherapy has even shown great promise against cancer. From my book, *Cancer: The Metabolic Disease Unravelled*:

Japanese researchers experimented with carbon dioxide for cancer in 2012 by directly injecting it into rat skin tumors at Kobe University School of Medicine. Published in the journal PLOS one, carbon dioxide injections were found to enrich cytochrome c oxidase activity, multiply the number of mitochondria in cells, trigger apoptosis in tumor cells and significantly reduce tumor volumes.

For dermatological and cosmetic purposes, modern research has confirmed that carboxytherapy stimulates blood flow, improves skin elasticity, has a necrotizing effect on fat tissue and reduces the appearance of cellulite. This came from a Czechoslovakian study in 2006 titled *Carboxytherapy—a New Non-Invasive Method in Aesthetic Medicine.*

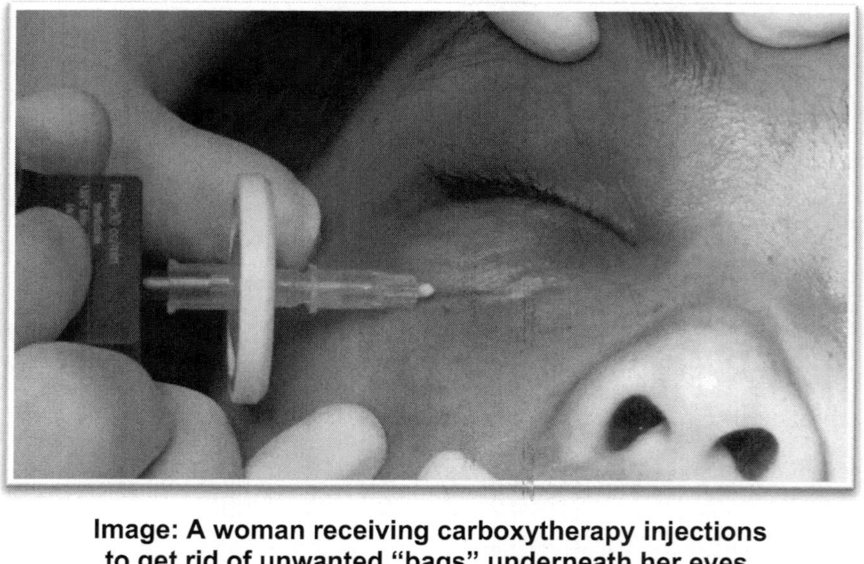

Image: A woman receiving carboxytherapy injections to get rid of unwanted "bags" underneath her eyes.

3. Carboxytherapy Gel

Good news for those of you who don't like being pricked with needles: Carboxytherapy can also be administered through the skin (transdermally) by applying a gel infused with carbon dioxide.

In recent years, a number of companies have brought products to market that contain carbon dioxide infused within gel, which can be applied to the body or on the face as a mask. Once applied, you simply wait a few minutes for the carbon dioxide to be absorbed and utilized for beauty and for health.

4. Carbon Dioxide Face Baths

Carbon dioxide face baths have become very popular in Japan and China. These involve filling a bowl with water, adding carbon dioxide, then holding your breath and dunking your face into it for as long as you can until you need to take another breath. This process can be repeated as many times as you'd like.

One way to add carbon dioxide to your face bath water is to purchase premade packets containing bicarbonate and an acid, which you mix into a bowl of water to carbonate it.

Another option is to buy a bottle of carbonated water (or a SodaStream® device) to carbonate your water and then dump it into a bowl for your face bath. Here's how a carbonated face bath looks…

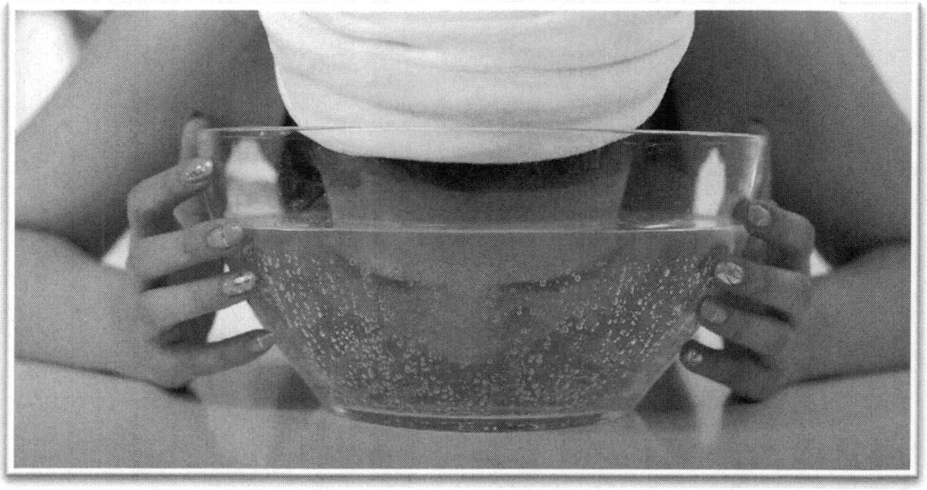

Image: YouTuber Tina Yong enjoying the invigorating experience of a carbonated face bath.

5. Drinking Carbonated Water

Speaking of carbonated water, at this point, it shouldn't be surprising to hear that *drinking* carbonated mineral water will have a therapeutic effect as well.

"Sparkling mineral waters of the 21st century are up-market drinks: Vichy, Evian, and Perrier persist as symbols of taste and class. More than just a drink, however, sparkling water represents one of the last vestiges of the therapeutic mineral springs that were a mainstay of Western medicine for more than two millennia," wrote Emily Pawley of the Science History Institute in an article titled *Powerful Effervescence.*

One of my absolute favorite types of mineral water that we have on shelves at grocery stores in my home province of Ontario, Canada is called *Gerolsteiner*. I have no affiliation with them; I just love their water and recommend you try it. If you are living in Germany, it'll probably seem like I'm preaching to the choir here since, according to their website, this naturally carbonated and mineral-rich beverage, which bubbles up through volcanic rock in Germany's Volcanic Eifel region, is "one of Germany's most-drunk mineral waters and No. 1 brand of sparkling mineral water in the world." A 1-liter bottle of this water is said to contain 1/3 of your daily calcium requirement and ¼ of your daily magnesium requirement.

That just about wraps up this chapter on carbon dioxide and its essential role in metabolism and its versatility as a therapy. I hope you found it useful.

Conclusions

Carbon dioxide baths have been used for thousands of years as a remedy for diseases of all kinds. The modern carbon dioxide or 'Nauheim' bath was named after the abundant carbonated mineral springs in Nauheim, Germany.

The carbon dioxide contained naturally in a carbonated mineral spring is the result of water bubbling up through volcanic rock and absorbing some carbon from it on its way to the surface.

Carbonated springs exist in many countries of the world including Europe and Japan, but in the United States and Canada, they are far less common. Saratoga, New York, California, and Idaho are among the few places in the United States that contain naturally carbonated springs.

Since most people can't afford to take the long and expensive voyage to Europe, American doctors came up with a solution that would allow patients who don't live near a carbonated mineral spring to still benefit from one: The "Artificial" (or simulated) Nauheim bath was born – and it quickly became the most popular therapy used by doctors in Western medicine for about a 100-year period until the 1940s.

In this chapter, you learned that when a cell is efficiently producing energy, within the mitochondria of every cell, in addition to copious amounts of ATP energy, a very important product is generated that keeps the metabolic rate high: carbon dioxide.

Carbon dioxide is the body's primary vasodilator, which increases the flow of blood throughout the entire body. It has anti-oxidant and anti-inflammatory properties and is essential for releasing oxygen from red blood cells for use in metabolizing energy. Everybody knows how important oxygen is – but without carbon dioxide, your body cannot use oxygen.

No matter which disease or symptom, when a person falls ill, their carbon dioxide levels will have dropped below the physiological norm – which indicates widespread cellular metabolic dysfunction.

By adding carbon dioxide back into the body of someone who is deficient in it, cells and tissues are suddenly able to breathe or 'respire' again in an upwards spiral that leads to the production of more carbon dioxide. Like giving a kid a push on his bike to get the wheels spinning, giving the body carbon dioxide will help it use oxygen, which will allow it to continue to metabolize efficiently on its own.

By adding sodium bicarbonate and an acid, or compressed carbon dioxide gas to a bath tub filled with water, one can create their own carbon dioxide bath at home. If you're adding CO2 to your bath via compressed gas, you'll know you've added enough when you see fine pearls of gas adhering to all your submerged skin. But before you do, ensure the water temperature is around 90° F to ensure the gas will dissolve in the water and not just bubble out of it.

Anybody who doesn't have access to a bath tub, or who wants to add more types of CO2 therapy to their regimen for beauty or for health, can also try dry carbon dioxide baths, carboxytherapy, carboxytherapy gel, carbon dioxide face masks, or sip on a carbonated beverage of their choice.

As science historian Emily Pawley wrote, "In sipping a glass of ginger ale, seltzer water, or Perrier, we are participating in a centuries-old tradition of therapy."

Key Points to Remember:

- Therapeutic use of carbon dioxide baths dates back thousands of years.
- The carbon dioxide bath is also called a Nauheim bath, named after the German town Nauheim, where carbonated springs are common.
- Carbon dioxide is absorbed into spring water from volcanic rock while bubbling up to the earth's surface.
- Simulated Nauheim baths were created in places like North America, where carbonated hot springs are rare.
- Nauheim baths were the primary remedy for disease in Western medicine for about 100 years beginning around 1835.
- Lack of oxygen is the primary cause of all chronic degenerative diseases; and carbon dioxide is essential for oxygen use.
- In all chronic diseases, there exists a deficiency in carbon dioxide.
- Administering carbon dioxide to sick patients appears to be the most efficient way to boost the body's metabolism.
- CO2 baths can be created at home by adding minerals like sodium bicarbonate and an acid to convert the ions of bicarbonate into carbon dioxide gas – and also by directly adding carbon dioxide from a compressed CO2 cylinder.
- Water temperature inside a carbon dioxide bath should be around 90° F and should not exceed 95° F.

CHAPTER 6

ENTER THE SIZZLER

This is it! You made it to the part of the book that some might call "the main event." This is the part where I tell you everything I know about bath bombs, including what they are and all the surprising benefits that I alluded to in the title of this book.

Most likely if you're reading this, you already know what a bath bomb is. It's a colorful and scented compressed ball of powder that you put in the bath tub to heighten your sensory experience.

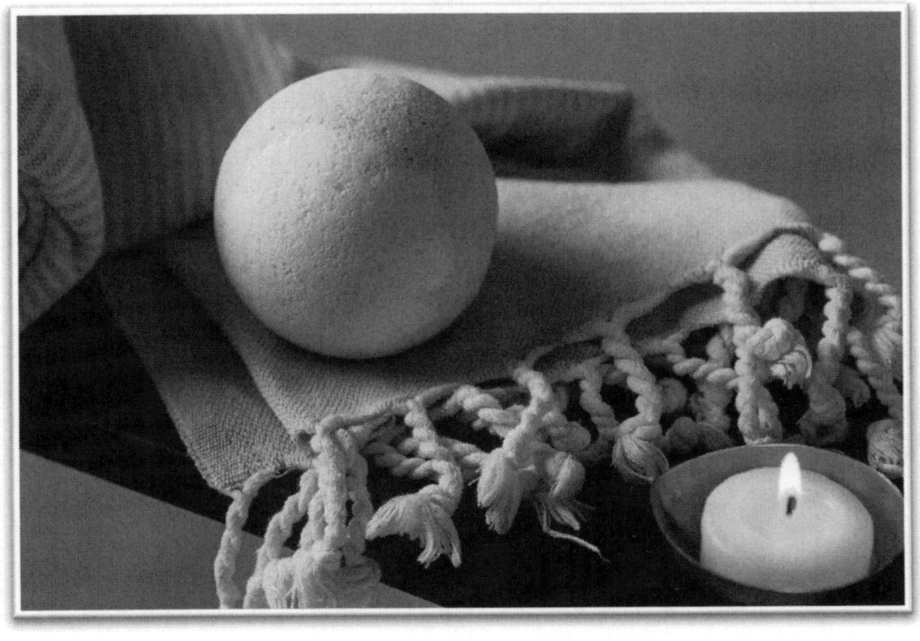

They're scented, fizzy, and fun – and when you drop one into water, a chemical reaction takes place that releases gas and causes the bath bomb to dissolve. But what is a bath bomb made of? What kind of gas does a bath bomb release? And what are the health benefits of bathing in a tub with a bath bomb dissolved inside? These are the questions I'm going to answer for you now.

The two active ingredients in a bath bomb that react together to release the medicinal gas are sodium bicarbonate and citric acid. If you haven't guessed already from reading the previous chapter on carbon dioxide, the gas that is produced is CO_2.

Sodium bicarbonate, also known as baking soda, is a type of salt that can be found in crystalline rock formations in nature. On a molecular level, sodium bicarbonate is the combination of sodium (salt) and bicarbonate, which is another form of carbon dioxide. Bicarbonate, the acid-neutralizing portion of sodium bicarbonate, is naturally produced by the human body and used to buffer excess acidity. It is a natural anti-bacterial, anti-viral and anti-fungal, which has been found to kill candida – the fungus responsible for yeast infections – as well as many other fungal strains that commonly infect human skin and nails. More than 90% of the carbon dioxide in your blood stream exists in the form of bicarbonate ($HC0_3$). The remainder of the CO_2 is either dissolved carbon dioxide gas (CO_2) or carbonic acid (H_2CO_3).

If you add baking soda alone to a bath, what you will get is water containing sodium ions and bicarbonate ions. But when you add an acid, the two compounds will react and the bicarbonate will be converted into carbon dioxide. This is the exact same thing that happens when you drop an Alka-Seltzer tablet into a glass of water. Interestingly, carbon dioxide is absorbed through your skin 100 times more powerfully than water.

Once dissolved inside water, the bath bomb begins to break apart – releasing all the colors, fragrances, salts and oils. Suddenly your bath water has become a silky smooth blend of psychedelic colors and scents.

If the water temperature is 95° F or lower, the carbon dioxide gas will be dissolved into the water in the form of carbonic acid. Every time you draw a bath and drop in a bath bomb, you're creating a carbonic acid bath.

Just like the formula Dr. John Harvey Kellogg used to create simulated Nauheim carbonated spring water for his patients at Battle Creek Sanitarium, bath bombs are a compact and simple way to carbonate your bath water.

Here is where things begin to get interesting. Since the key player here is sodium bicarbonate, let's get into the many uses and health benefits of baking soda.

Health Benefits of Baking Soda

For most people, baking soda is nothing more than a box of white powder that they put in the fridge to neutralize smells caused by leftover food or juice that was spilled on one of the shelves. If you're one of those people, you will probably be quite surprised to hear that hospitals routinely infuse sodium bicarbonate solutions into patients intravenously as an antidote for chemical poisonings – and that sodium bicarbonate can make you a better athlete.

Exercise Performance Enhancement

You'll recall from the chapter on carbon dioxide the study I presented in which swimmers who soaked in carbonated water as a warm-up before swimming had significantly increased red and white blood cells during their swim and significantly reduced changes in heart rate and blood lactic acid content after their swim. A similar study has been done on athletes soaking in water containing a bath bomb prior to swimming.

After their bath bomb-infused warm-up soak, the Japanese athletes performed swimming tests and the scientists analyzed various parameters of their metabolism and performance. Results showed that swimmers who underwent carbon dioxide baths prior to swimming had improved muscle performance, increased endurance, and accumulated lower levels of lactic acid during their swim.

You might be surprised to hear that many more studies have been conducted on the impact of sodium bicarbonate for athletic performance. Research has shown that orally consumed sodium bicarbonate can...

- Increase back squat repetitions to failure
- Improve 200m swimming time
- Significantly increase punches landed during four rounds of boxing
- Improve cycling performance during repeated sprints
- Again, all of those benefits were obtained through consuming as much as 2 tablespoons of baking soda orally, which in my experience, is absolutely disgusting. Another issue with consuming it orally is that it can cause stomach upset in large doses.
- By hopping into your bath tub and dissolving a bath bomb inside, you will obtain all the performance-enhancing CO2 you need without having to force foul tasting powder down your throat.

Detoxification

"If you want to see how fast a person can hit the floor during chemotherapy, just forget to mix in the bicarbonate and get out your stopwatch!" exclaimed Dr. Mark Sircus in his book *Sodium Bicarbonate*. Yes, oncologists regularly administer sodium bicarbonate solutions intravenously to cancer patients before injecting chemotherapy in their veins to protect them from the deadly poison because sodium bicarbonate is incredibly effective at neutralizing and helping the body to detoxify chemical poisons.

Doctors in hospital emergency rooms routinely use intravenously-injected bicarbonate for chemical poisonings of all kinds, including herbicides glyphosate and paraquat, yew berry poisoning, and uranium poisoning. Sodium bicarbonate is also an effective remedy for people who have overdosed on prescription drugs, like Amitriptyline or Flecainide. In people who have overdosed on anti-depressant drugs or crack cocaine, intravenous sodium bicarbonate can be used to eliminate their seizures and restore heart rate abnormalities to normal.

But, of course, no needles are necessary in order for us to get the carbon dioxide needed to detoxify our bodies of the myriads of toxic chemicals which we are exposed to on a daily basis. Dissolving a bath bomb in the bath tub and soaking our bodies in the life-giving water will do the trick.

Fat Loss

Have you ever noticed that as you age it becomes increasingly easier to put on weight and increasingly more difficult to lose it?

That's because your metabolic rate is generally highest at birth and will steadily decline over the course of a lifetime right up until the point of death in old age. Maintaining the highest metabolic rate that you can is the key to safe and lasting weight loss. The higher your metabolic rate, the more energy your body will burn at rest in any given unit of time – and the more energy your body burns at rest, the less likely you will gain weight and the easier it is to lose weight.

Many people believe the popular myth that jogging for an hour every day will raise their metabolism because they're burning more calories. But the reality is jogging and endurance exercise is very stressful on the body and typically lowers metabolism. One of the reasons for this is hyperventilation, which wastes valuable CO2 in the exhaled breath. If somebody who is constantly lowering their basal metabolic rate through jogging ever stopped jogging, it will be easier than ever for them to put on fat.

When the metabolism falls, your rate of calorie burning decreases and your body begins to manufacture more fat out of the food you eat. The stress from a low metabolic rate causes increased triglycerides in your blood, which leads to insulin resistance, increased fat storage, and other hallmarks of obesity and metabolic syndrome.

Any food, practice, or therapy that can boost your metabolism will help you lose unwanted fat – and this is exactly what sodium bicarbonate can do for you. American researchers investigated the impact of an intravenous infusion of sodium bicarbonate solution on cellular metabolism in 1956. The study reports that the infusion stimulated respiration and increased metabolic rate, as evidenced by ☒o☒an increased output of CO2."

Environmental Remediation

Industrialization and the use of toxic chemicals in pesticides, food packaging, electronics, paints, fabrics, furniture, and other common products means that our exposure to toxic chemicals is at an all-time high. These same chemicals make their way into waterways like streams, rivers, lakes and oceans, polluting all plant and animal life they come in contact with. We've got a lot of work to do to remediate the damage that has been done.

People implementing regenerative practices on their permaculture farms are doing enormous good for the environment by eliminating the use of pesticides, completing the water cycle and recharging aquifers, and using ruminant animals to quickly rebuild topsoil that has been lost from agriculture.

But what about all the chemicals released into the environment? There's hope for that too. Amazingly, sodium bicarbonate can help us detoxify not only our bodies, but also our environment.

Research has found that sodium bicarbonate can help us clean chemical pollutants out of both soil and water. Sodium bicarbonate can…

- Neutralize high aluminum concentrations in water
- Remove 92% of uranium from contaminated soil samples
- Remove polychlorinated biphenyl (PCB) from waterways
- Clean one metric ton of PCB-tainted soil per hour in a rotary reactor

Isn't it good to know that every time you take a bath with one of your favorite bath bombs inside, you're also helping cleanse the environment by sending one of nature's safest and most powerful detoxifying agents down the drain?

Cancer

Anybody who hasn't lost someone to cancer at this point is lucky. As cancer rates continue to climb, ignorance is no longer an option, so listen up:

In the 1930s, Dr. Otto Warburg showed that cancer cells were simply cells that lost their ability to utilize oxygen. Cancer is a disease of impaired cellular respiration.

When the cell loses its ability to oxidize glucose within the mitochondria, it reverts to a more primitive type of cell metabolism called anaerobic glycolysis – which is the conversion of glucose into lactic acid. This is why all cancer patients have an excess of acidity in their bodies.

Dr. Leonard Coldwell, author of *The Only Answer To Cancer*, has spoken about the fact that all cancer patients will have excess acidity in their body, called lactic acidosis – and that once the blood is alkalized, the cancer growth stops. He mentions a number of ways to neutralize the acidity, including the consumption of alkaline foods, like fruits and vegetables. Grass fed dairy is another food containing an abundance of alkaline minerals and is the highest source of calcium of all foods. What else do we have in our toolbox that can neutralize acids?

The sodium bicarbonate in bath bombs and the CO2 that it produces can be used to switch off the production of lactic acid and restore oxygen use inside cells. This is why sodium bicarbonate can be useful for cancer.

Make no mistake about it, your doctor or other people working in the medical industry will probably tell you that sodium bicarbonate is a 'quack treatment' that has no medical value. They will probably even try to scare you away from it by claiming that it's dangerous. But these are some of the easiest claims in the world to prove wrong. Should we be surprised that an industry which generates $126 Billion a year would feel threatened by an effective remedy that costs about $1?

Dr. Coldwell has stated that in his experience, through alkalizing the blood of cancer patients, "Every cancer can be cured in two to 16 weeks." Aside from his direct clinical experience working with cancer patients, there has been quite a lot of scientific research testing sodium bicarbonate on cancer. The following is from my book titled *Cancer: The Metabolic Disease Unravelled*:

Dr. Robert J. Gillies and his team from the H. Lee Moffitt Cancer Center & Research Institute in Florida examined the relationship between tumor microenvironment pH and the growth and spread of cancer in vivo. Results were published in the journal *Cancer Research* in 2013 and found that oral administration of sodium bicarbonate inhibited the growth and spread of colon and breast tumors. "In every case, the regions of highest tumor invasion corresponded to areas of lowest pH. Tumor invasion did not occur into regions with normal or near-normal extracellular pH," they wrote. In other words, an acidic tumor environment is essential for cancer metastasis and balancing out the pH using sodium bicarbonate can prevent it from occurring.

One of the mechanisms behind the anti-metastatic effect of sodium bicarbonate was discovered by scientists Ian Robey and Lance Nesbit from the University of Arizona in 2013. Their study found that sodium bicarbonate reduced the number of circulating tumor cells in the blood of tumor-bearing mice to less than half.

Dr. Gillies and his team discovered another mechanism behind sodium bicarbonate's anti-cancer effects in 2016. It is well established that excess acidity impedes immune system function and that neutralization of acidity with sodium bicarbonate can amplify the immune response. After administering sodium bicarbonate to tumor-bearing mice, the researchers observed an influx of immune cells into tumors, which prevented the growth of numerous tumor types.

The controversial claims made by Dr. Leonard Coldwell and others advocating the use of sodium bicarbonate for cancer are validated by this research. If you're interested in learning more, my book *Cancer: The Metabolic Disease Unravelled* contains hundreds of studies on the use of sodium bicarbonate for cancer, as well as a number of testimonials from people who have used it successfully – even after doctors told them there was nothing more they could do and sent them home to die.

Baking soda is one of the cheapest and most effective remedies ever discovered ⊠ttt and soaking in a bath tub with a bath bomb dissolved in it is one of the easiest and most pleasant ways to receive the medicine.

Essential Oils in Bath Bombs

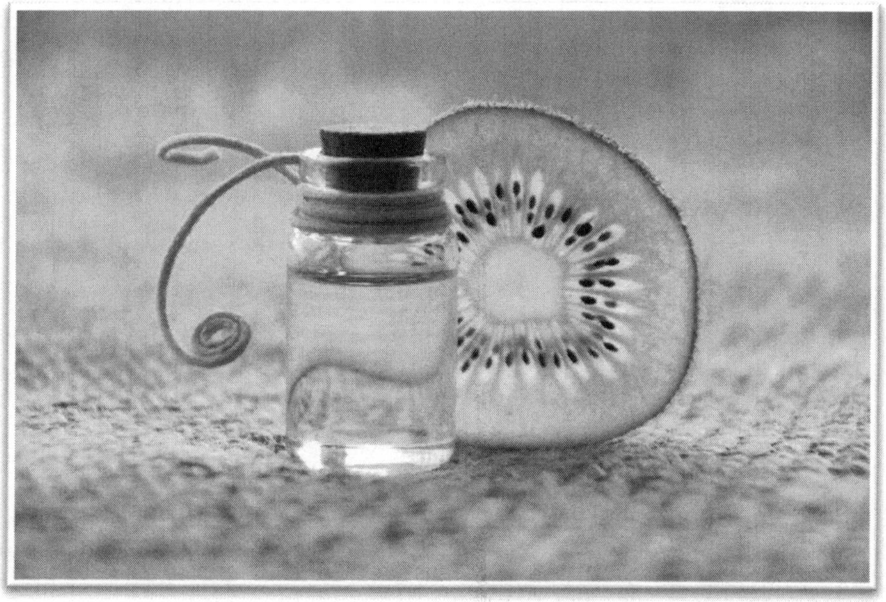

Many commercially-produced bath bombs contain one or more types of essential oils, which can add flowery fragrances or other plant aromas to the bath tub. Some of the most popular essential oils today include mint, ginger, lemon, orange, grapefruit, jasmine, lavender, chamomile, rose and cinnamon. But what are essential oils, and do they have any health benefits?

Essential oils are the oils extracted from a plant. They are "essential" in that they contain the fragrant essence of that plant. The oils often contain hundreds of aromatic compounds, some of which have positive health effects and some have negative.

Given the fact that there are literally thousands of different plants that you could gather essential oils from, each of which contain their own assortment of chemical compounds, talking about all of it is beyond the scope of this book. But here's a brief overview of essential oils so you have an idea what they are, what they might be able to do for you and which ones you should probably avoid.

Since the middle ages, essential oils have been widely used for bactericidal, virucidal, fungicidal, antiparasitical, insecticidal, medicinal and cosmetic purposes, and there's lots of recent scientific studies validating most if not all of those applications. Some studies show inhaling essential oils like lavender before bedtime can help you sleep. And according to a 2014 review on essential oils, "Their anticancer activity is well documented."

Despite the published science, it's interesting to note there are many "hit pieces" coming from the mainstream media in recent months that warn against the use of essential oils. For example, an article appeared in *The Huffington Post* in February 2020 titled "Sorry, your essential oils are essentially useless." Could this misinformation be the handiwork of the pharmaceutical industry in attempts to funnel money away from the billion dollar essential oil industry and back into their pockets? Sounds like a good business move to me. Whether that's the case or not, it doesn't seem to be working. A recent poll by Insider found that 1/3 of Americans believe in the health benefits of essential oils and aromatherapy. Because essential oils are nothing more than pure extracts from plants, people tend to have very strong intuition that these natural products are good for them.

However, I must mention that just because something comes from a plant doesn't mean it's good for you.

7 of the World's Deadliest Plants

"They may look harmless enough, but plants can harbor some of the most deadly poisons known. From the death of Socrates by poison hemlock to the accidental ingestion of deadly nightshade by children, poisonous plants have been responsible for human deaths throughout history," writes Melissa Petruzzello in an article on *Britannica*.

If anybody ever offers you essential oils from the following seven deadly plants, be sure to run the other way:

1. Water Hemlock
2. Deadly Nightshade
3. White Snakeroot
4. Castor Bean
5. Rosary Pea
6. Oleander
7. Poison Ivy

There are deadly plants, and then there are plants that probably won't kill you (unless you consumed a huge amount of them) but overall have a negative impact on your health. Phytoestrogens are chemicals contained within certain plants which mimic the stress hormone estrogen. Before I list some phytoestrogen-containing plants, here's a quick lesson on the physiological effects of estrogen in the body:

The famous 1990's Women's Health Initiative study tested the effects of supplemental estrogen on women, but the trial was forced to stop early after participants began developing cardiovascular disease, stroke, dementia, and cancer.

7 Plants containing Phytoestrogens

The following is by no means a complete list of estrogenic plants, but here are some of the most common that you'll want to avoid eating, and also avoid putting their essential oils in your tub:

1. Chasteberry
2. Licorice
3. Hops
4. Soy
5. Black cohosh
6. Red clover
7. Dong quai

If you really love the scent of any of those plants and want to add some essential oil to your bath bomb, I say go for it – the carbon dioxide will protect you to a great degree. However, bathing in estrogenic plant oils everyday might not be a good idea.

Another horrible idea is buying bath bombs that contain toxic chemical ingredients.

Warning: Toxic Dyes and Chemicals in Bath Bombs

Unfortunately, ingredient toxicity is an issue that spans industry wide in the world of cosmetics, and it appears bath bombs are no exception.

Lush makes "the original fizzy bathtime treats" – but just because they invented the bath bomb doesn't mean their bath bombs are safe. I must admit they have some of the most exuberant and wacky spheres of kaleidoscopic bath treats I have ever seen – and with names to match! But as I look at the list of ingredients on their labels, I can say with certainty that you'll never find them in my bath tub.

Take their bath bomb *Mermaid Tail* for example. It contains a number of different essential oils like lemon myrtle oil and Ylang Ylang oil and even some organic skin conditioners like cocoa butter, which are highly beneficial.

However, the list of ingredients I don't want anywhere near me is a lot longer than the ones I do, and it includes a lot of words that are difficult to pronounce like sodium laureth sulfate, fragrance, synthetic fluorphlogopite, titanium dioxide, laureth 4, sodium coco-sulfate, cocamidopropyl betaine, tin oxide, calcium sodium borosilicate, alpha-isomethyl ionone, hydroxycitronellal, ultramarines, blue 1, iron oxides, blue 1 lake, green 3, red 28, yellow 5.

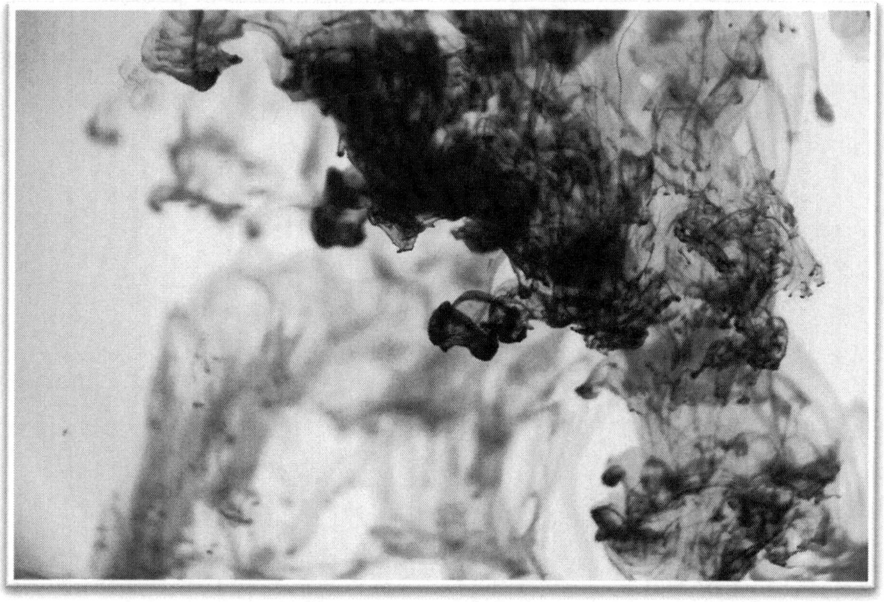

Every single one of these chemical compounds is foreign to the body, and they will all likely disrupt your body's metabolism and function of every organ and system governed by your metabolism, such as immunity, hormones, digestion, etc. Replacing personal care products that are toxic with ones containing clean ingredients is an act of self-love.

Anybody looking for clean bath bombs will be happy to know that many great companies on the market today are producing organic bath bombs. They're great if you don't have the time to make your own bath bombs and also great to give to friends and family as gifts. Next birthday or holiday, buy someone you love this book and a bath bomb or two and watch their eyes light up. The bath bombs and salts I recommend can be found, along with a 10% discount code at the following page: https://www.endalldisease.com/store/

But why buy bath bombs when they're easy, fun and inexpensive to make?

How to Make a Bath Bomb

Making bath bombs is not difficult. With a few bucks and an hour of your time you can literally make yourself enough bath bombs to last you a few months.

All the funkadelic shapes aside, here is what you need to create a bath bomb that you can use to carbonate your next bath.

- 1 cup of baking soda
- ½ cup citric acid
- ½ cup cornstarch
- Methylene blue
- 1 bath bomb mold

Instructions:

First, mix the 1 cup of baking soda, the ½ cup of citric acid and ½ cup cornstarch together into one bowl. All three of those items are available at your local grocery store.

Next, add 1 teaspoon of water to your mixture, which should barely moisten the mix and cause it to stick together.

And lastly, scoop the mixture into a mold. This can be any mold you like – from a classic spherical bath bomb mold to a star-shaped candy mold. The best place to find molds are at craft stores and sometimes bulk food stores. Of course, Amazon has lots of these molds as well. Whichever mold you choose, keep the mixture in the mold overnight until it dries – and *voila*! Just like that you're done.

Healthy Blue Dye?

You may have heard of an inexpensive blue dye called methylene blue. It's safe, beautiful, and will make your bath *even more* medicinal. Methylene blue is often used in fish tanks to keep fish healthy but it's also a remarkable metabolic remedy for humans. It works similarly to red light therapy by photodissociating nitric oxide bound to a critical respiratory enzyme within the mitochondria of your cells called cytochrome c oxidase. All that scientific mumbo jumbo is to say methylene blue is a safe yet powerful enhancer of cellular metabolism.

And all you bath lovers seeking more beautiful skin will be happy to hear that methylene blue has an anti-aging effect on skin. A 2017 study in the journal *Nature* called methylene blue "a traditional mitochondrial-targeting antioxidant" which "improved skin viability, promoted wound healing, and increased skin hydration and dermis thickness." Methylene blue is "safe for long-term use, and did not cause irritation even at high concentrations," concluded the researchers.

You're welcome.

CHAPTER 7

7 PRINCIPLES OF THE ULTIMATE HEALING BATH

In the 19th and early 20th centuries, when balneotherapy was the primary therapy in Western medicine, Dr. John Harvey Kellogg created a formulation which he believed would be of the greatest benefit for his patients at Battle Creek Sanitarium. However, science has advanced significantly since that time – so we're going to take the opportunity to improve upon his formula and make one that's even better.

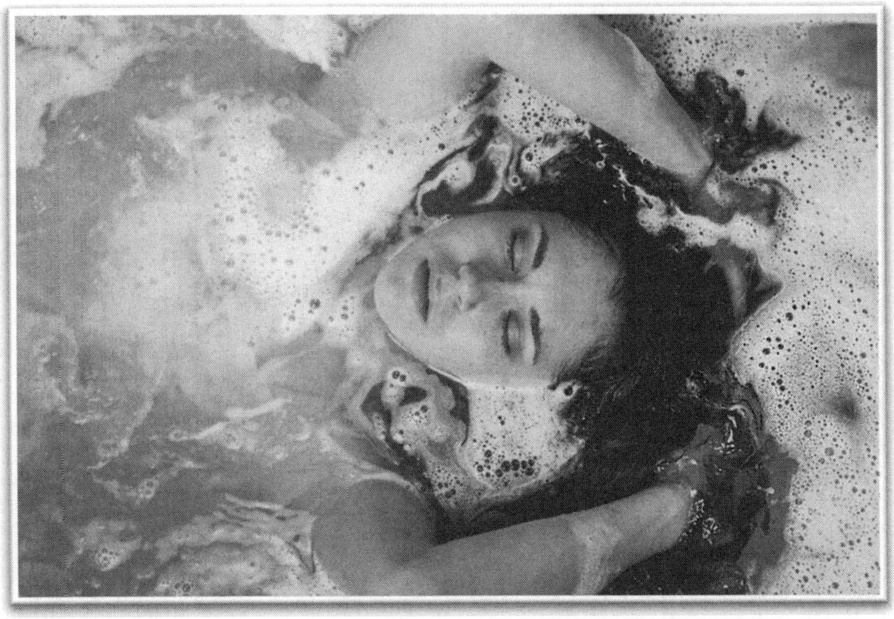

Dr. Kellogg's formulation was developed *before* the work of Dr. Maynard Murray, which showed us the incredible mineral profile of ocean water and the remarkable impact that being exposed to these minerals can have on our health. Dr. Kellogg's formulation was also developed *before* the physiology of carbon dioxide was understood. It was even developed before mitochondria and the process of oxidative phosphorylation were discovered. (For the record, Mitochondria were discovered and named by Carl Benda in 1898). This explains why the benefits of bathing in carbonated waters were a mystery to doctors at that time – they simply knew it worked. What's my point in saying all this?

My point is that, through our investigative work in this book, we've determined an evidence-based bath formulation that far exceeds the healing potential of the bath formulations used by even the most elite doctors of the 19th and 20th centuries. I've gathered seven principles that I'll outline for you now.

Revelations

The therapeutic aspects that we've investigated in this book include temperature, mineral content, and carbon dioxide content. Now it's time for a synthesis of all that information so we can render everything down into a simple formulation that will serve to enhance our metabolisms to the greatest possible degree.

Below is the list of each principle that we will use to unlock the door to the ultimate therapeutic bath.

Ultimate bath principle #1: Hot water increases metabolic rate/ cold water decreases it

The temperature of your body directly corresponds to how well your metabolism is working. You can't have a low temperature and a high metabolic rate. When your temperature drops below the ideal 98.6° F, your metabolic rate will also drop with it. And by elevating your body temperature back up to 98.6° F, your metabolic rate will also increase.

Ultimate bath principle #2: Hot water detoxifies heavy metals and other environmental chemicals

Most people don't associate a hot bath with an activity that results in massive amounts of sweat being released because you can't see droplets of sweat while your entire body is immersed in water. When you bathe in warm or hot water, the sweat released will result in the detoxification of heavy metals and other environmental contaminants from your body.

Ultimate bath principle #3: Hot water absorbs more dissolved minerals than cold water

One of the principles that you may have learned in high school chemistry class is the greater the water's temperature, the greater its capacity for dissolving minerals or other solids. We see this in the warm waters of the Dead Sea, which is usually very warm, depending on the time of year, and contains as much as 10x more mineral solids than the cooler waters of the ocean.

Ultimate bath principle #4: Dehydrated ocean minerals contain every necessary soluble mineral in the *exact* proportions your body needs

Due to rainfall and runoff stripping minerals from land on its journey to the sea, ocean water contains over 90 water-soluble minerals and trace elements, all of which the body needs and in *exact proportions* required by the blood serum of humans, animals, and other biological life. As a result, cancer does not exist in sea creatures, according to the work of Dr. Maynard Murray. It's clear that dehydrated ocean minerals as well as minerals from the Dead Sea are the ultimate base mineral mixture to add to your bath tub.

Ultimate bath principle #5: The ideal temperature range for a carbon dioxide bath is 86-95° F

Unlike minerals, which are absorbed in greater amounts as the water temperature increases, gases are absorbed into water better as the temperature is reduced. Doctors in the 19th century hydrotherapy clinics knew this, and that's why they generally kept the water temperature of carbon dioxide baths between 85 and 95° F. This temperature range seems worth repeating as it's a good middle ground where water is satisfactorily carbonated while still comfortable for bathing.

Ultimate bath principle #6: Minerals prevent CO2 from escaping the bath water

Another important discovery that can help us prevent carbon dioxide escaping from our bath water came from the lifeB⊠⊠5⊠s work of Dr. Simon Baruch. Baruch taught us that the addition of minerals to a carbonated bath will prevent that carbon dioxide from leeching out of the water, compared to water absent of minerals.

Ultimate bath principle #7: Minerals help the body absorb more CO2

The other major discovery of Dr. Simon Baruch that has helped us with our bath formulation is that adding minerals to carbonated bath water will increase the skin's absorption of carbon dioxide. Adding minerals to our CO2 bath will benefit us in at least three ways – the benefit of the minerals themselves, by preventing CO2 from escaping the bath water, and by helping our skin absorb more CO2.

Synthesis

We've now established the key principles that will allow you to create the most therapeutic bath you can possibly make right in the comfort of your very own bath tub at home.

Using these principles, we can distill down a simple bath formula to add to your bath tub. Make sure your water is 90° F and add the following ingredients:

- 1-2 lbs. Ocean minerals
- 1-2 lbs. Epsom Salts

- 1 or more Bath bombs/Carbon dioxide gas
- 1-10 drops of Essential Oil
- 1-50 drops of Methylene blue

Instructions:

Ocean salts

Adding 1-2 lbs. of ocean minerals to your bath water will provide your body every mineral it needs in perfect proportion. Like the cancer-free whales and other aquatic creatures, you'll soon be wading in a brine containing zero mineral deficiencies. Your body will absorb the minerals and use them as needed to resolve chronic mineral deficiencies that you may have had for your entire life.

Epsom salts

Epsom salts are available at most pharmacies and yet most people walk by not knowing their body is screaming for the minerals contained in those bags of salt. Epsom salts are magnesium sulfate. Around 70% of people are deficient in magnesium and a large number of people are also deficient in sulfur. This is why you may have heard of people raving about bathing in sulfur springs. Unless you're eating foods fertilized with ocean minerals or grown in soil amended with ocean algae or sea vegetable compost, you're likely deficient in magnesium and sulfate. Adding 1-2 lbs. of Epsom salts to your bath tub will infuse these valuable minerals into the water.

Bath bombs/Carbon dioxide gas

Adding one or more bath bombs to the tub will infuse your bath water with nourishing CO_2. Some people may want to skip the bath bombs and directly inject CO_2 into their bath with a pressurized cylinder. Attach an aquarium diffuser stone to the end of the hose and bubble the CO_2 into the water until you see silver bubbles form on your skin. Whichever method you choose, carbonating your bath water is the foundation of your bath. Make sure you carbonate your bath *after* you add your ocean minerals and Epsom salts, since the minerals will prevent CO_2 from escaping out of the water.

Essential oils

Adding 1-10 drops of your favorite fragrant botanical oils to your bath tub is the perfect way to pamper another one of your senses for a richer, more aromatic experience while making the bath water more therapeutic. Avoid oils from plants containing phytoestrogens and the oils will synergize with the carbon dioxide, minerals and temperature for an even more potent experience.

Methylene Blue

The medicinal yet inexpensive blue dye known as methylene blue is a great addition to the bath tub to color it with a beautiful blue while fortifying your water with another safe and potent metabolic medicine. Adding 1-50 drops of methylene blue to your tub will add beauty to stimulate even more of your senses for a more holistic experience while igniting a therapeutic synergy within the water.

Session Time

How long should you bathe in your CO_2 bath each session?

Common and effective session times for CO_2 baths range from 10 to 30 minutes, with all the remarkable results you're looking for. But bathing in carbonated water for up to an hour might even be more beneficial.

In one study mentioned earlier in this book, on athletic performance of Japanese swimmers, a quick 20 minute carbonated bath, resulted in "better performance during swimming and less accumulation of fatigue-related metabolites after swimming." The improved swimming performance and reduced fatigue-related metabolites are good indicators that the CO_2 is being absorbed and utilized within that time frame.

At the end of the day. nobody knows your body better than you. I encourage you to experiment with different session times, within the range of 20 minutes to an hour, then take note of how you feel after, until you find what works best for you.

Add Some Light

One of the best ways to supercharge your balneotherapy sessions with curative power is to lay in the sun – with as much skin exposed as possible – for about 15-30 minutes, either before or after your bath. Some hot springs and seas like the Dead Sea exist outside in the open air, and these two treatments have traditionally gone hand-in-hand. When you combine balneotherapy with light therapy (phototherapy), you get the longest word that either of us have probably read all day: balneophototherapy.

Everybody knows that the sun emits UV light which is essential for the production of Vitamin D. But if you've read my book *Red Light Therapy: Miracle Medicine,* you'll know that around 60% of the light emitted from the sun is in the red and near-infrared range, which is in many ways *even more* beneficial than the vitamin D-producing UVB. As Dr. Ray Peat once said, "Red light is probably the primary anti-stress factor for all organisms."

Here are a few additional studies you might be interested in about balneophototherapy:

- "The addition of phototherapy to balneotherapy, or balneophototherapy, further enhances the anti-inflammatory effects of thermal spring water." https://pubmed.ncbi.nlm.nih.gov/29908578

- Balneotherapy + UVB light therapy is superior to UVB light therapy alone for treating psoriasis https://pubmed.ncbi.nlm.nih.gov/17714121

- Baths with the thermal waters of Comano Springs, Italy plus UVB phototherapy was effective in 94% of psoriasis patients. https://pubmed.ncbi.nlm.nih.gov/2609852

And if you're one of those people who are afraid of the sun, don't be. As long as you're not getting burnt, exposure to sunlight is virtually pure benefit. Lay on your stomach in your bathing suit, set the timer for 15 minutes, and lay there until your alarm sounds. Then, flip onto your back and repeat before heading inside for a soak in your bath tub to complete your balneophototherapy session.

Experimenting with Ingredients

We've now established the formulation for the most therapeutic bath you can possibly make right in your very own bath tub at home. However, one of the things that's not an exact science is the amount of each ingredient to add. The amount of ocean minerals, Epsom salts, bath bombs, essential oils and methylene blue I've listed above will be an excellent formulation for most people and you'll never have to worry about changing it.

But for the experimental types, I encourage you to experiment by increasing or decreasing the concentration of minerals, carbon dioxide, essential oils and methylene blue you add to your baths. And there is even a way to track your progress and how much CO2 your body has obtained from each bath.

Measuring CO2 Changes with a Capnometer

Any increase in carbon dioxide in your blood means an increase in your body's metabolism. And it turns out the amount of carbon dioxide in your exhaled breath is an accurate indicator of the amount of CO_2 in your blood.

For those who want to see exactly how well the baths are working for them, you can use a device called a capnometer, which you breathe into to measure the changes in carbon dioxide in your exhaled breath before, during, and after your baths.

At the time of writing this, I haven't found any capnometers on the market that I would recommend; most of them are way overpriced and don't provide features like graphing changes in your breath. That's why a friend of mine – the same man who developed the CO_2 dry bath suit and CO_2 sauna – is developing a capnometer that will actually track changes in your CO_2 in real time and graph them for you. This device can be used to see *in real time* the precise metabolic changes that occur in your body from each bath. By the time you're reading this, the product may be available, so be sure to check the store page on Endalldisease.com if you're interested.

Conclusions

Using principles gathered from the research and experience of elite doctors of the 19th and 20th centuries, as well as scientific research that has occurred since that time, we've established a bath formulation that far exceeds the healing potential of the bath formulations of the past. Furthermore, it also likely far exceeds the therapeutic potential of bathing in the ocean, the Dead Sea, or any natural hot springs in the world.

The healing baths in which we soak, based on the 7 principles I've established in writing this book, undoubtedly rank high among the greatest remedies available to us.

Anybody who sees through the limitations of the toxic drug- and surgical-based medical industry in this world will be thrilled at these new developments and eager to get started.

In order to help you get started, I've created a *Carbon Dioxide Therapy Email Course* exclusively for people who've purchased this book to guide you step-by-step on how to get the proper tools and ingredients needed to begin CO2 baths and other forms of carbon dioxide therapy in all its forms quickly, safely, and easily. I'll leave a link for you to sign up on the very last page of this book.

With a glass of Gerolsteiner naturally-carbonated mineral spring water in my right hand, I propose a toast to your health and mine. *Cheers!*

RECOMMENDED RESOURCES

Sea Energy Agriculture by Maynard Murray

The Cure (1917) short film by Charlie Chaplin
https://www.youtube.com/watch?v=Sqx6iz6_UJ8

Image attributions

Soda springs Geyser:
https://commons.wikimedia.org/wiki/File:Soda_Springs_Geyser_2.JPG

Battle Creek Sanitarium:
https://commons.wikimedia.org/wiki/File:Battle_Creek_Sanitarium_with_tower.jpg

CO2 cylinder and bath tub:
https://commons.wikimedia.org/wiki/File:Rational_therapy_(1919)_(14589535479).jpg

ABOUT THE AUTHOR

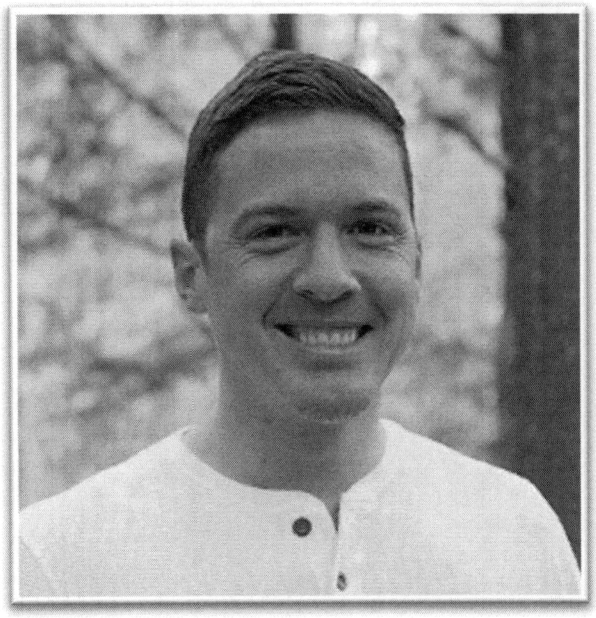

MARK SLOAN has written over 300 articles and is the author of *The Cancer Industry*, *Cancer: The Metabolic Disease Unravelled* and the 6x international #1 bestseller *Red Light Therapy: Miracle Medicine*. Mark lives in Ontario, Canada and his goal is to build an off grid home, raise a big, beautiful family and live a self-sufficient, resilient and responsible life as God had intended. Mark is passionate about learning and his ultimate goal in life is to reduce the suffering in this world and to make a better place for every human being alive and for future generations.

PLEASE REVIEW THIS!

I hope you enjoyed this book and found the information valuable. Above all, I hope it gives you hope for a brighter future.

If this book helped or entertained you in any way, all I ask in return is that you take a moment to write an honest, sincere review of this book on Amazon. It will only take a few minutes, and it will help me out more than you can imagine.

To leave a review, search "Bath bombs Mark Sloan" on Amazon to find the book page or visit the following link, then scroll down and write a couple of quick sentences:

amazon.com/dp/1777239605

MORE INTERNATIONAL #1 BESTSELLING BOOKS BY THE AUTHOR

- The Cancer Industry
- Cancer: The Metabolic Disease Unravelled
- Red Light Therapy: Miracle Medicine
- The Ultimate Guide to Methylene Blue
- Bath Bombs & Balneotherapy
- And more!

Checkout all of Mark Sloan's books by visiting the following link:

ENDALLDISEASE.COM/BOOKS

THE BEST BATH BOMBS IN THE WORLD!

Find out which premium quality bath bombs and bath salts I use and get a discount code for 10% off your purchase at the link below.

- Premium quality bath bombs
- Mineral salts infused with amino acids and eucalyptus
- Made in the USA
- Support a small family business

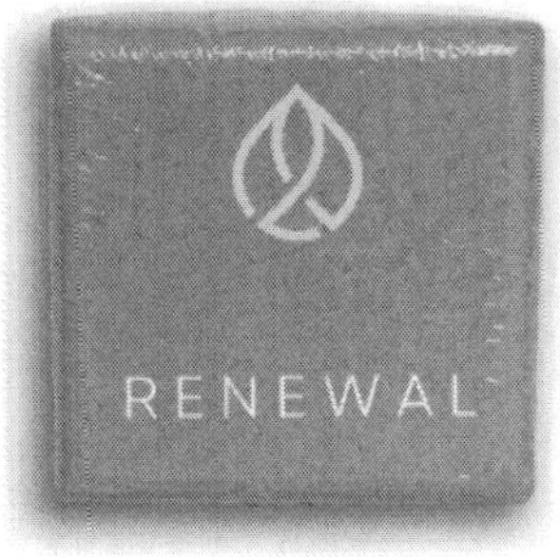

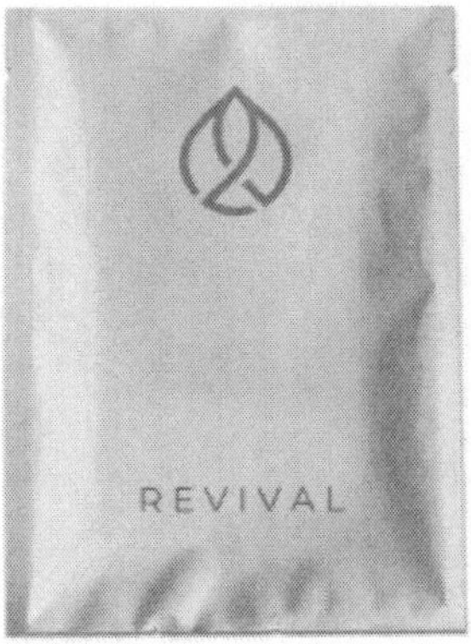

Visit the link below:
Endalldisease.com/balneotherapyunlockdiscount

FREE GIFT #2: RED LIGHT THERAPY VIDEO COURSE

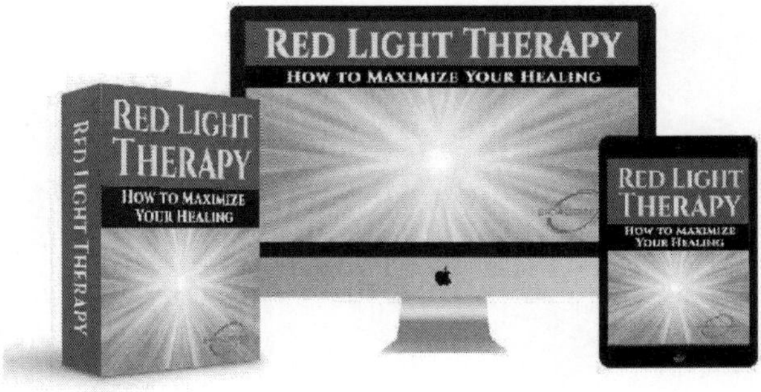

Want to know what Red Light Therapy can do for your health and how to get remarkable results from home?

Watch the world's first Red Light Therapy Video Course by #1 Bestselling Author of Red Light Therapy: Miracle Medicine, for FREE at the link below:

ENDALLDISEASE.COM/SPECIALOFFER

FREE GIFT #3: INSIDER DEALS

Get the world's most powerful metabolic therapies and technologies for your medicine cabinet at home – at a discount!

Unlock exclusive Endalldisease Insider deals on red light therapy, methylene blue, balneotherapy, hormone therapy, CO2 therapy, and more, for FREE at the link below:

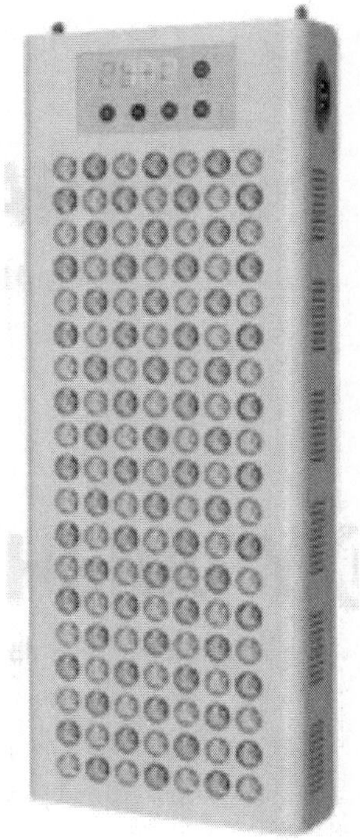

Endalldisease.com/unlockdiscounts

Printed in Great Britain
by Amazon

35362704R00068